1 MONTH OF
FREE
READING

at

www.ForgottenBooks.com

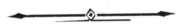

By purchasing this book you are eligible for one month membership to ForgottenBooks.com, giving you unlimited access to our entire collection of over 1,000,000 titles via our web site and mobile apps.

To claim your free month visit:
www.forgottenbooks.com/free979494

ISBN 978-0-260-87647-8
PIBN 10979494

NOTES

ON

THE EYE,

FOR THE USE OF

UNDERGRADUATE STUDENTS,

BY

FRANK LARAMORE HENDERSON, M. D.

PROFESSOR OF OPHTHALMOLOGY IN THE BARNES MEDICAL COLLEGE, ST. LOUIS
MO.; OPHTHALMIC SURGEON TO ST. MARY'S INFIRMARY, THE CENTENARY HOS-
PITAL AND THE CHRISTIAN ORPHANS HOME; CONSULTING OCULIST TO THE
WABASH RAILWAY, AND TO THE TERMINAL RAILWAY ASSOCIATION;
MEMBER OF THE AMERICAN MEDICAL ASSOCIATION; MEMBER OF
THE MISSOURI STATE MEDICAL ASSOCIATION; VICE-PRESIDENT
OF THE ST. LOUIS MEDICAL SOCIETY, AND SECRETARY
OF THE ST. LOUIS MEDICAL LIBRARY ASSOCIATION.

SECOND EDITION.

ST. LOUIS, MO.:
NIXON-JONES PRINTING CO.
1900.

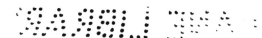

PREFACE.

The students' manuals on diseases of the eye, which I have seen, are either exhaustive treatises in fine print or condensations of the *entire* science of ophthalmology. The authors of these works seem loath to omit any knowledge which, as specialists, they have acquired. The result is that subjects which the general practitioner never attempts to master are given as much space as those with which he should be familiar.

It should be the purpose of a medical school to provide its graduates with an equipment which will best meet the demands of general practice, and I recognize that there is enough matter to fill the course to overflowing, that is of more importance than the layers of the retina or the formula for calculating the index of refraction of a transparent medium.

The only claim to originality made for this work lies in its omissions. Minute anatomy, optics, the fitting of glasses, skiascopy, ophthalmoscopy and kindred subjects have been left out intentionally, as I believe they belong to post-graduate instruction. I have also slighted those diseases which have to be diagnosed with the ophthalmoscope, as I doubt the diagnostic value of an ophthalmoscope in the hands of the average general practitioner.

It is not my desire to minimize medical education but rather to increase the *useful* knowledge of the graduate by selecting that which will be of the most service to him, at the same time giving him as much as the undergraduate student can reasonably be expected to learn in the limited time allotted to the eye in our medical schools. The use of these printed notes enables the teacher to devote much time to quizzing which would otherwise be spent in lecturing, and the medical student will agree with me that it requires rare and peculiar talents to make of a medical lecture anything but a dreary recital of facts. This book also enables the student to dispense with his inaccurate and misleading classroom notes. The subject has been divided into twenty-four lessons, or one lesson for each week of a six months' session. In the spelling of such words as oxid, quinin, morphin, sulfate, etc., the rules adopted in 1891, by the American Association for the Advancement of Science, have been followed.

CENTURY BUILDING,
St. Louis, Mo.

CONTENTS.

LESSON I.

ANATOMY OF THE EYE.

THE ORBITS.

These four-sided, pyramidal or conical cavities, a little over an inch and a half deep, are formed by seven bones: frontal, sphenoid, ethmoid, superior maxillary, palate, malar and lacrymal. On the inner wall of the orbit is the groove, formed by the lacrymal bone and the nasal spine of the superior maxillary, in which is lodged the *lacrymal sac.*

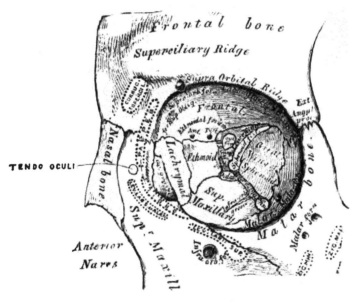

FIG. 1.—Left orbit. (Gray.)

In front of this groove is the insertion of the orbicularis, the muscle which closes the eyelids, and behind the groove is the insertion of the tensor tarsi or Horner's muscle which holds the lids close to the globe. In the angle formed by the roof of the orbit and the nasal wall, and a short distance behind the orbital rim, is the loop or pulley through which passes the tendon of the superior oblique muscle. In the angle formed by the roof and the temporal wall and just under the edge of the orbit is a fossa which holds the lacrymal gland. At the junction of the inner and middle thirds of the superior orbital rim is the *supra-orbital notch* or foramen through which passes the supra-orbital nerve, artery and vein. Below the infra-orbital rim is the *infra-orbital foramen*, which is the termination of the canal of the same name. Near the apex of the orbit and between the great and lesser wing of the sphenoid bone is the *sphenoidal fissure*, which transmits the third, fourth, the ophthalmic division of the fifth and the sixth nerves and the ophthalmic vein. The apex of the orbit corresponds to the *optic foramen*, a cylindrical canal in the lesser wing of the sphenoid bone, which transmits the optic nerve and ophthalmic artery.

Extending forward and outward from near the apex is the *spheno-maxillary fissure*. It lies between the lower border of the great wing of the sphenoid bone and the maxillary bone, and transmits the infra-orbital vessels and several nerves. In the middle of the orbital floor is the *infra-orbital groove* which terminates in the *infra-orbital canal*. The bones are covered by periosteum and the orbital space not filled by the eyeball, nerves, muscles and vessels, is occupied by fat and connective tissue. This connective tissue becomes thickened in parts so as to form sheaths for the muscles and optic nerve. It also develops a membrane which spreads over the eyeball, from the entrance of the optic nerve to within three millimetres of the cornea where it becomes inseparably mingled with the conjunctiva. This membrane is called *Tenon's capsule*. It is loosely connected to the episclera, the space between them serving as a lymph channel. The *ophthalmic artery*, a branch of the internal carotid, supplies blood to the orbit and its contents.

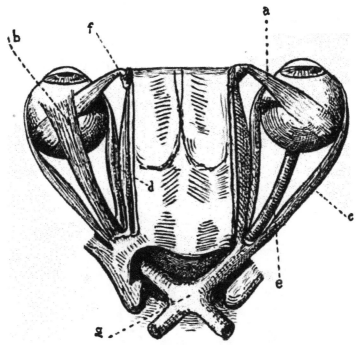

FIG. 2. — The ocular muscles seen from above. a, Superior oblique; b, Superior rectus; c, External rectus; d, Internal rectus; e, Optic nerve; f, Pulley of superior oblique; g, Optic commissure.

THE OCULAR MUSCLES.

The ocular muscles are six in number, the internal, external, superior and inferior recti, and the superior and inferior oblique. All except the inferior oblique arise from the apex of the orbit around the optic foramen. The inferior oblique arises from the floor of the orbit in a slight depression in the superior maxillary bone near the lacrymal groove. All the ocular muscles, after piercing the capsule of Tenon are inserted in the sclera, the four recti at points varying from 5.5 to 7.5 millimetres from the cornea.

Though the superior oblique arises at the apex of the orbit, the direction of its force is changed by passing through the pulley, before mentioned, which is situated in the angle formed by the roof and the nasal wall of the orbit. From this pulley its direction is backward and outward and passing under the superior rectus, it is inserted into the outer side of the globe, more than half of the tendon being inserted back of the equator. The inferior oblique runs backward and outward, and passing between the orbital floor and the inferior rectus, it is inserted into the outer side of the globe, more than half of the tendon being back of the equator at a point below the superior oblique.

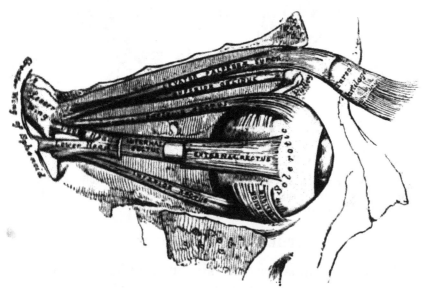

FIG. 3.— Muscles of the right eye. (Gray.)

In addition to its scleral attachment, some fibres from the superior rectus and its sheath pass to the conjunctival fornix and to the top of the tarsus, by which means these structures are moved in harmony with the upward movement of the eyeball. The termination of the inferior rectus is similar to that of the superior. In the same way fibrous bands are given off from the sheaths of the internal and external recti and pass laterally to the bones and soft parts of each side of the orbit. The *levator palpebrae superioris* muscle, which lifts the upper lid, owing to its location, is best described with the ocular muscles. It arises at the apex of the orbit and passes forward just under the roof of the orbit to its insertion into the top of the superior tarsus by a fan-shaped aponeurosis, which is as broad as the lid itself. The motor muscles of the eye are supplied with blood by the muscular branches of the ophthalmic artery. The external rectus muscle is supplied by the *sixth* nerve, the superior oblique by the *fourth* nerve, and the four remaining motor muscles, as well as the levator palpebrae superioris, by the *third* nerve.

THE LIDS.

Under the skin of the lids is a thin layer of connective tissue, and under this the fibres of the *orbicularis muscle*. The orbicularis, which closes the lids, may be divided into a palpebral part which lies in the lids proper and an orbital portion which mingles with the muscles of the forehead and cheek. The former arises from the internal palpebral ligament, the latter from the bones in front of the lacrymal groove. The *tensor tarsi*, or Horner's muscle, which is sometimes considered a part of the orbicularis, arises from the lacrymal bone behind the groove. Both of these muscles are supplied by the portio dura of the seventh or facial nerve. Under the orbicularis are *the tarsi*, formerly called cartilage, now known to be dense fibrous tissue. There is one of these thin, flat, elongated plates in each lid to give it form and support, the tarsus of the upper lid being twice as wide as the tarsus of the lower. The tarsi are connected at their extremities and also bound to the subjacent bone by the internal and external palpebral ligaments. These ligaments are thickened fibres of a circular fascia, the *septum orbitale*, which extends from the rim of the orbit to the orbital edge of the tarsi. Under the tarsi and in groves in their substance are the *Meibomian glands.*

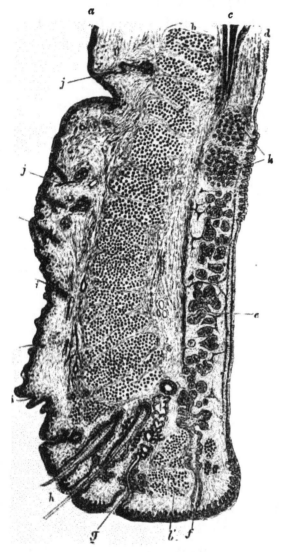

Fig. 4. — Vertical section through the upper eyelid. (Schafer.) a. Skin; b. Orbicularis; b'. Ciliary bundle; c. Involuntary muscle of eyelid. d. Conjunctiva; e. Tarsus; f. Meibomian gland; g. Sebaceous gland, or gland of Moll; h. Eyelashes; i. Small hairs in skin; j. Sweat gland; k. Lacrymal lobules.

They number about thirty in the upper and twenty in the lower lid. They resemble currants on a stem, the stem

lying across the tarsus and at right angles to the edge
of the lid. Their ducts open on the free margin of
the lid. They are sebaceous glands, and the fluid they

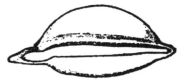

FIG. 5.—The tarsi. (Schwalbe.)

secrete prevents adhesion of the lid borders. Under the
Meibomian glands is the conjunctiva, the mucous membrane which covers the inner surface of the lids. The
opening between the lids is called the *palpebral fissure*.

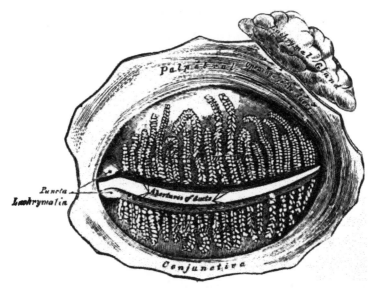

FIG. 6.— Position of Meibomian glands, the conjunctiva removed. (Gray.)

The nasal end of the fissure is the *inner canthus*, the temporal end is the *outer canthus*. The eyelashes are arranged in two rows and their follicles are supplied with
sebaceous glands, near which are found the glands of Moll,
usually described as modified sweat glands.

LESSON II.

ANATOMY OF THE EYE (*Continued*).

THE LACRYMAL APPARATUS.

The lacrymal apparatus is divided into the secretory part and the excretory part. The former is composed of:
1. The *lacrymal gland*, which is lodged in a fossa at the upper and outer angle of the orbit. It is about the size of the kernel of an almond, and the fluid it secretes (tears) empties into the conjunctival sac near the superior temporal fornix through small tubes, six to ten in number.
2. A large number of glandular *lobules* identical in structure and function with the lacrymal gland, imbedded in the loose connective tissue of the conjunctival fornix, and also found in the tarsi near their orbital borders. These lobules are largest and very much more numerous in the upper lid at the external canthus, which has led to their description in this region as the inferior or palpebral lacrymal gland.

The excretory apparatus begins with the four minute openings: the *puncta*, one of which is located on each lid border about a quarter of an inch from the inner canthus. The puncta open into small tubes, the *canaliculi*, which empty by a common orifice into the side of the *lacrymal sac* at a point just behind the internal palpebral ligament. The sac extends upward two or three millimetres above the internal palpebral ligament and is continuous below with the *nasal duct*, which empties into the inferior nasal fossa. The total length of the sac and duct is about one inch. Their direction is a little backward and outward from the vertical.

THE CONJUNCTIVA.

The conjunctiva is a mucous membrane. Its e_itielial layer rests u_on the membrana _ro_ria w_ici is com_osed of w_ite fibrous and elastic tissues. The membrana _ro-_ria is united to the underl_ing structures b_ a la_er of sub-mucous connective tissue. There is considerable variation in the _istolog_ of the three _arts w_ici the conjunctiva _resents for examination.

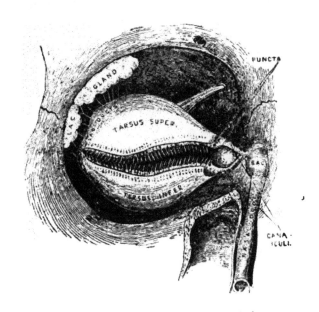

FIG. 7.—The Lacrymal apparatus. (Juler.)

1. The *palpebral* conjunctiva lines the inner surface of the lids. It is slightly velvet_, due to numerous fine grooves and _its in its surface; the elevations between the grooves are called *papillae*. The membrana _ro_ria is closely ad_erent to the tarsus, and in it are said to be found numerous l_mp_oid follicles.

2. The *ocular* conjunctiva covers the anterior t_ird of the eyeball exce_t the cornea. Histologically the outer layer

of the cornea is similar in structure to that of the scleral conjunctiva but clinically they appear so different that it is confusing to a student to describe the conjunctiva as covering the cornea. The ocular conjunctiva is very loosely connected to the underlying tissues except at the circumference of the cornea where it adheres firmly. On the ocular conjunctiva, near the inner canthus, is a round, fleshy body, an accumulation of glandular follicles called the *caruncle*, and just external to the caruncle is the *plica semilunaris*, a fold of the conjunctiva which is the analogue of the third eyelid of some animals.

3. The ocular and palpebral portions above described are connected by a loop or fold of mucous membrane called the conjunctival *fornix*. In the fornix are located the glandular lobules which may be considered accessory lacrymal glands.

In the conjunctiva is a considerable plexus of lymphatic vessels, which communicate with the lymph spaces of the cornea. The blood supply is from branches of the ophthalmic, facial and internal maxillary. The sensory nerves come from the lacrymal and nasal branches of the first division of the fifth nerve.

THE EYEBALL.

The eyeball is a globular body a little less than one inch in diameter. It is not quite a perfect sphere, as the anterior segment, the cornea, has a greater curvature than the rest of the globe. Anatomists are not agreed as to which diameter is the longest.

The real difference in the size of the eyes of individuals is much less than the apparent difference. The apparent difference being due to the position of the ball in the orbit, whether set forward or far back, and to the shape of the lids and the width of the palpebral fissure. Normally the eye should be so placed that a line drawn from the upper to the lower orbital margin would just touch the cornea.

The eyeball consists of three coats or tunics:—

1. The external, fibrous coat, composed of the sclera and cornea.

2. The middle coat, called the uveal tract, composed of the choroid, ciliary body and iris.

3. The nervous coat, the retina.

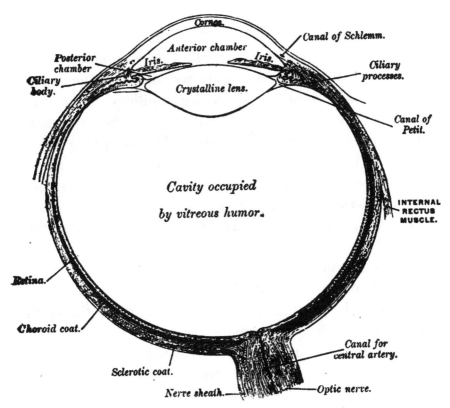

FIG. 8. — A horizontal section of the eyeball. (Allen.)

The interior of the eye is divided by the crystalline lens into the aqueous and vitreous chambers.

The aqueous chamber is divided by the iris into an anterior and posterior chamber.

The following terms are useful for descriptive purposes :—

The *axis* of the eye is a line drawn from the center of the cornea, through the center of the ball, to a point between the optic nerve and macula lutea. The corneal end of this line is the *anterior pole*, the other end, the *posterior pole* of the eye. A circle around the ball at an equal distance from the poles is the *equator*. Other circles around the ball, passing through the poles, are *meridians*.

THE CORNEA.

The cornea is the transparent, glassy-looking, circular membrane which forms the anterior sixth of the eyeball. It has no blood vessels except the capillary loops which encircle its periphery and encroach upon its substance a distance of about one millimetre. The nutrition of the cornea is, in great measure, supplied by lymph derived from this capillary system, though the deeper layers derive some nourishment from the fluid of the anterior chamber by osmosis. The nerve supply is from the fifth and is very profuse.

The cornea has five layers : —

1. In front a layer of *epithelium*, six to eight cells deep, which is continuous with and similar to the epithelium of the scleral conjunctiva.

2. The anterior limiting layer or *membrane of Bowman*, a homogeneous, apparently structureless, resisting layer, which is supposed to be the most instrumental in maintaining the normal corneal curve. It is with difficulty separated from the substantia propria.

3. *Substantia propria* or proper substance of the cornea, a transparent fibrous tissue, not as dense as the preceding, forming the greater part of the thickness of the cornea. It is composed of about sixty layers, the

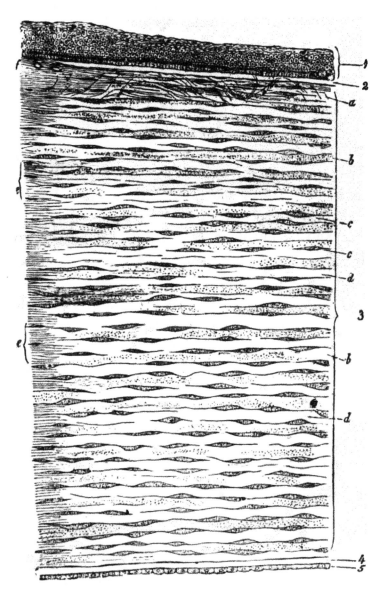

FIG. 9.—Section of cornea near the limbus. (Schafer.) 1, Epithelium; 2, Bowman's membrane; 3, Substantia propria; 4, Descemet's membrane; 5, Endothelium; a, Oblique fibres in the anterior layer of the substantia propria; b, Lamellae the fibres of which are cut across, producing a dotted appearance; c, Corneal corpuscles appearing fusiform in section; d, Lamellae the fibres of which are cut longitudinally; e, Transition to the sclerotic, with more distinct fibrillation, and surmounted by a thicker epithelium; f, Small blood vessel cut across near the margin of the cornea.

fibres in each running in the opposite direction to the fibres in the layer above and below. Between these layers are found cell spaces which communicate with each other and serve as lymph channels. Within the cell spaces are found the corpuscles, the connective tissue cells of the cornea.

4. Posterior limiting layer or *membrane of Descemet,* a thin, homogeneous, brittle layer, the most resisting of the cornea.

5. A single layer of *endothelial* cells. This layer covers the ligamentum pectinatum at the angle of the anterior chamber, and is continued over the anterior surface of the iris.

ANATOMY OF THE EYE (*Continued*).

THE SCLERA.

The sclera composes five sixths of the outer tunic of the eyeball. It is made of white fibrous and yellow elastic tissue with some pigment in its deeper layers. It is essentially of the same constituents as the cornea, but its tissues are so arranged as to almost wholly intercept rays of light. Though the sclera is tough and resisting, the form of the eye is not maintained by it, as it will collapse if the contents of the ball escape.

The sclera is covered by a thin layer of loose connective tissue called the *episclera*. The optic nerve passes through the sclera at a point about 3 millimetres toward the nasal side and 1 millimetre below the posterior pole of the ball. It does not enter in one bundle but divides and passes through numerous openings. This sieve-like part of the sclera is called the *lamina cribrosa*. Around the lamina cribrosa the numerous posterior ciliary vessels and nerves pierce the sclera. Behind the equator the 4 to 6 venae vorticosae find their exit, and about 2 millimetres from the cornea the 5 to 8 anterior ciliary arteries pass in to their distribution to the iris and ciliary body. The sclera and underlying choroid are connected by a very loose, pigmented connective tissue, whose meshes communicate so as to form a lymph space: the *perichoroidal*. If the sclera is separated from the choroid half of the brown, pigmented connective tissue adheres to the sclera forming its inner layer, called the *lamina fusca*. The contents of the perichoroidal space escape through lymph channels which are found around the vessels and nerves that pierce the sclera. The sclera is poorly supplied with blood vessels, its nourishment coming mostly from the lymph of the perichoroidal and periscleral spaces. Completely encircling the cornea, but lying in the scleral tissue, is found the *canal of Schlemm*. There is yet a division of opinion as to whether it is a venous or lymphatic channel. That it is instrumental in draining the anterior chamber is generally accepted.

THE IRIS.

From a point corresponding to the internal junction of the cornea and sclera a curtain is suspended in the aqueous chamber. This curtain, the iris, is the most anterior portion of the uveal tract or vascular coat of the eye. It is composed of muscular fibres, pigment, blood vessels, nerves and connective tissue. The amount of pigment in the iris determines its color, which may vary from the pink of an albino to the deep brown of a negro. In the center of the iris is a round opening: *the pupil*. The muscular fibres of the iris are involuntary (unstriped) and are divided into radiating and circular fibres. The latter are arranged around the pupil and act as a sphincter in contracting it. These fibres are controlled by the *third* nerve. The radiating fibres are supposed to dilate the pupil and are controlled by the *sympathetic* nerve. The function of the iris is to regulate the amount of light entering the eye. In accomplishing this its action is reflex, the afferent nerve being the optic, the efferent nerve the third. In front of the iris and between it and the cornea is the *anterior chamber*. The region of the anterior chamber where the cornea and iris unite is called the angle of the anterior chamber. In the angle of the anterior chamber is found the *pectinate ligament*, composed of interlacing trabeculae, which extend from Descemet's membrane of the cornea to the iris. The sponge-like framework of the pectinate ligament incloses numerous intercommunicating spaces: *the spaces of Fontana*. Behind the iris is the *posterior chamber*. Viewed laterally (meridional section), the

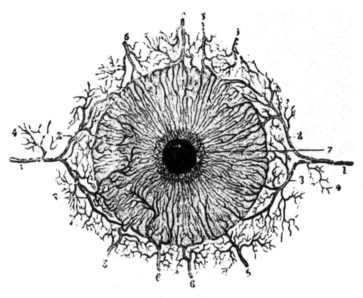

FIG. 10. — Arteries of the iris. (Sappey.) 1, 1, long posterior ciliary arteries; 2, 3, their branches of bifurcation; 4, recurrent arteries destined for the choroid; 5, 5, 6, 6, anterior ciliary arteries anastomosing with the long ciliary to form the greater arterial circle of the iris; 7, the lesser arterial circle of the iris.

posterior chamber is triangular in shape. The base of the triangle is the ciliary body; the two sides, the iris and lens; the apex, the point where the pupillary margin of the iris comes in contact with the lens. The anterior and posterior chambers form the *aqueous chamber*. The long ciliary arteries, two in number, arise from the ophthalmic and pierce the sclera, one on each side of the optic nerve. They pass forward between the choroid and sclera to the periphery of the iris, where they divide into an ascending and descending branch. The six to eight anterior ciliary arteries are derived from either the muscular or lacrymal branches of the ophthalmic and pierce the sclera near the corneal junction. They anastomose with the branches of the long ciliary to form the *circulus arteriosus iridis major*, from which branches radiate toward the pupil and around its margin form the *circulus arteriosus iridis minor* (Fig. 10).

THE CILIARY BODY.

The ciliary body lies between the iris and the anterior end of the retina. It is firmly adherent to the sclera at the anterior end but loosely attached behind. It is divided into two parts : —

1. The *vascular* part, which is composed of convoluted blood vessels, connective tissue and pigment, lies next to the vitreous and supplies it and the lens with much of their nourishment. It is also supposed to be the principal agent in the secretion of the aqueous humor. The anterior part of the vascular portion is thrown into seventy or eighty projecting tips, the *ciliary processes*.

2. The *muscular* part lies next to the sclera and is the agent of accommodation. Its fibres are unstriped and are arranged in two sets. Those nearest to the sclera run meridionally and those next to the iris equatorially. Contraction of the ciliary muscle is produced by those fibres of the ciliary nerves which are derived from the third. The long ciliary nerves, two or three in number, are given off from the nasal nerve which is a branch of the ophthalmic; the ophthalmic being the first division of the trigeminus or fifth. The short ciliary nerves, ten or twelve in number, arise from the *ciliary* or *lenticular ganglion*. This ganglion, which is about the size of a pin head, is found back of the globe between the optic nerve and external rectus muscle.

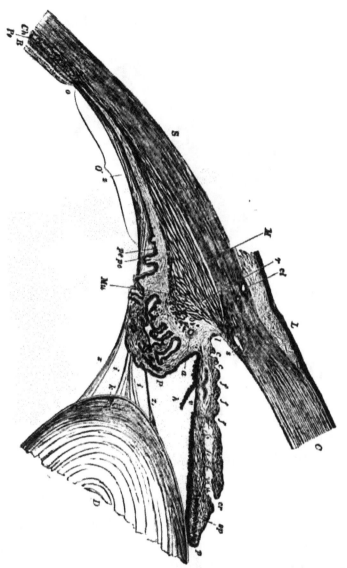

FIG. 11.—Section through the ciliary region. (Fuchs.) C, cornea; S, sclera; Ch, choroid; R, retina; Pe, its pigmented epithelium; o, orra serrata; O, pars ciliaris retinae; this is continued over the ciliary processes; pe, pe, pigmented and non-pigmented cells of pars ciliaris; D, lens; M, ciliary muscle; r, its radiating fibres; Mu, circular fibres; ci, anterior ciliary artery; S, canal of Schlemm; z, origin of ciliary muscle; e, e, f, f, folds and depressions in anterior surface of iris; cr, a crevice in this surface (? artificial); sp, sphincter pupillae; p, edge of pupil; P, most prominent part of ciliary process; h, pigment behind iris, detached at v; a, blood vessel; z, zonula of Zinn; z', z', its continuation or the suspensory ligament; i, i, spaces between the fibres of the suspensory ligament; k, capsule of lens.

It is supplied by three roots from the fifth, third, and sympathetic nerves. The long and short ciliary nerves pierce

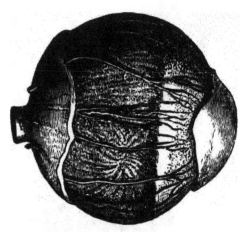

FIG. 12.—The sclera removed, showing the ciliary nerves, passing through the suprachoroidal space to reach the anterior part of the eye (after Merkel).

the sclera around the optic nerve and pass forward between the choroid and the sclera to the ciliary muscle and iris (Fig. 12).

THE CHOROID.

Extending from the ciliary body back to the optic nerve and lying next to the sclera is a vascular membrane, the choroid. It is connected to the sclera by the loose fibrous trabeculae described on page 15. It has four layers.

1. When the sclera and choroid are torn apart half of this fluffy, pigmented membrane adheres to the sclera (lamina fusca) and half to the choroid. The part adhering to the choroid is called the *suprachoroidea*. It is reddish-brown in color, due to the presence of numerous stellate, pigmented cells.

2. Under the suprachoroidea is found the *lamina vasculosa*, a layer of arteries and veins held together by connective tissue. There are also some stellate pigment cells

in this layer. The arteries are derived from the twelve to twenty short posterior ciliary, which arise from the ophthalmic and pass through the sclera around the optic nerve. Some recurrent branches from the long ciliary and the anterior ciliary arteries enter into the anterior portion of the lamina vasculosa.

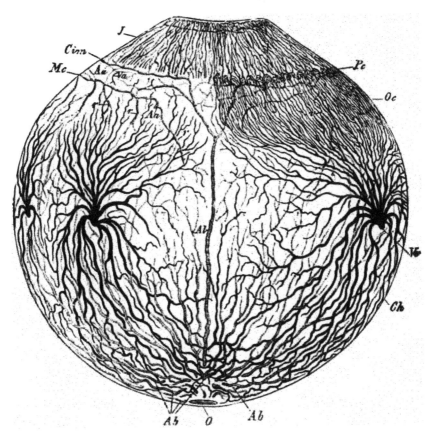

FIG. 13.—Circulation of the choroid. (Leber.) O, optic-nerve entrance; Oc, ciliary region; Pc, ciliary processes; J, iris; Aa, anterior ciliary arteries; Ab, short posterior ciliary arteries; Al, long posterior ciliary; Cim, circulus arteriosus iridis major; Mc, arteries of ciliary muscle; Vv, vena vorticosa.

3. The arteries divide and anastomose to form a capillary layer under the lamina vasculosa called the *choriocapillaris*. The chorio-capillaris helps to nourish the retina

and vitreous. The veins of the choroid arise from the chorio-capillaris and from the ciliary body and iris and unite into four or six groups. Each group empties near the equator through one vein, the *vena vorticosa*. The venae vorticosae empty into the ophthalmic vein.

4. Under the chorio-capillaris and firmly united to it is found the innermost layer, the *lamina basilis*. It is a thin transparent layer of condensed connective tissue.

LESSON IV.

ANATOMY OF THE EYE (*Continued.*)

THE LENS.

Behind the iris and in contact with its pupillary margin lies the crystalline lens, a circular, biconvex, transparent body, composed largely of albumen and water. Its posterior surface fits into the hyaloid fossa of the vitreous.

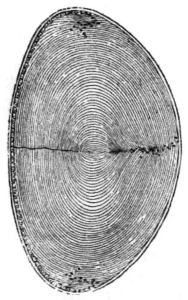

FIG. 14. — Meridional section through the crystalline lens. (Babuchin.)

The curvature of the posterior surface is much greater than that of the anterior. The lens is contained in a transparent capsule, named according to location the *anterior* and *posterior* capsules. The peripheral edge, or the point of union between the anterior and posterior capsules, is called the *equator* of the lens.

The lens is held in position by the suspensory ligament, or *zonula of Zinn*, which is composed of delicate fibres that arise from the posterior surface of the ciliary processes. These fibres are inserted into the equatorial region, some going to the anterior and some to the posterior capsule. The lens is divided into a dense central part, the *nucleus* and a softer peripheral part, the *cortex*. There is no abrupt transition between these parts, there being a gradual centrifugal increase in the density of the lens as age advances.

THE VITREOUS.

The interior of the eyeball, back of the lens, is filled by a transparent, jelly-like substance, the vitreous, which maintains the shape of the eye, and holds the retina and lens in position. It has no blood vessels or nerves and is nourished by lymph from the vessels of the ciliary body, retina and choroid. Through its center from the optic disc to the center of the posterior surface of the lens, runs the *hyaloid canal*, a lymph channel, which is supposed to communicate in front with the aqueous humor and behind with the lymph spaces surrounding the optic nerve. In fetal life it contains the hyaloid artery. The vitreous is contained within a thin capsule, the *hyaloid membrane*. Anteriorly the vitreous presents the *hyaloid fossa* into which the posterior surface of the lens fits.

THE RETINA.

The fibres of the optic nerve pass through the lamina cribrosa and spread between the choroid and vitreous, forming an almost transparent membrane, the retina. It extends forward to a point corresponding with the union of the choroid and ciliary body, terminating in a wavy line called the *ora serrata*. It is composed of ten layers, the most external or one lying next to the cioroid, being a pigment layer wiici does not terminate at the ora serrata but continues over the ciliary body and ,osterior surface of the iris to the margin of the ,u,il.

The otier nine layers are com,osed of very com,licated nerve structures and tieir su,,orting connective tissue. In the center of the retina is a round area about one twentieth of an inci in diameter, the *macula lutea*, so called from the yellow color it assumes soon after deati. In the center of the macula is a sligit de,ression wiici a,,ears as a more dee,ly colored ,oint or s,ot. Tiis s,ot, wiici corres,onds to the ,osterior end of the visual axis, is called the *fovea centralis*. It is the center of direct vision and the most sensitive ,art of the retina. A little toward the nasal side of the retina is seen the large, circular wiite s,ot, the *optic disc* or intra-ocular end of the o,tic nerve. The arteria centralis retinae ,ierces the o,tic nerve 1.5 centimetres from the eyeball and ,asses forward tirougi its center to the o,tic disc where it divides into its brancies, wiici s,read out in all directions in the retina. Tiere is no anastomosis between the retinal arteries, ience an obstruction of one of tiem results in destruction of the area wiich it nourisies. The retinal veins lie by the side of the arteries. The retina is attacied to the underlying structures only at the optic disc and at the ora serrata. Sirinkage of the vitreous is ,rone to cause se,aration of the retina from the cioroid anywhere between tiese two ,oints.

THE OPTIC NERVES.

An o,tic nerve may be divided into tiree ,arts: 1. Intra-ocular. 2. Orbital. 3. Intra-cranial.

1. The o,tic nerve fibres ,ass tirougi the sclera at the lamina cribrosa and tien radiate in every direction to form

the retina. That portion of the nerve between the lamina cribrosa and the point where it disperses to form the retina is called the head of the nerve, the *optic disc* or optic papilla. With the ophthalmoscope it shows as a round white spot almost in the center of the posterior wall of the eye. (See colored plate.)

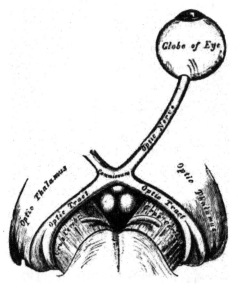

FIG. 15.—Optic tracts and commissure. (Bowman.)

2. The orbital portion of the optic nerve extends from the sclera to the optic foramen. It curves in the shape of an S, which enables the eye to move freely in all directions without subjecting the nerve to undue tension. The nerve fibres, about half a million in number, are collected into numerous bundles which are inclosed in a framework of connective tissue. The sheaths of the optic nerve are three in number, the dura, arachnoid and pia mater, which originate from the same membranes of the brain. Under the dural sheath is a lymph space: the subdural, and under the arachnoid another: the sub-arachnoid space. These spaces communicate with the cerebral spaces of the same name. Anteriorly, the three sheaths merge into the sclera.

3. The intra-cranial portion of an optic nerve extends from the optic foramen to the chiasm, a distance of less than one centimetre. In this region it has lost its two outer sheaths which have merged into the corresponding membranes of the brain. Though the optic nerves proper end at the chiasm, their fibers are conveyed from the chiasm to their termination in the brain by two nerve bundles called the *optic tracts*. In the chiasm or *optic commissure*, which lies in the optic groove of the body of the sphenoid bone, a partial decussation of the optic nerve fibres takes place.

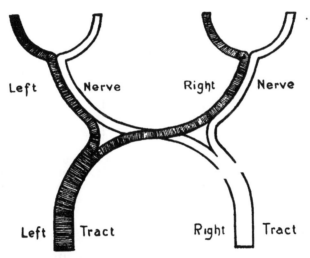

FIG. 16.—Decussation of the optic nerve fibres.

The fibres from the nasal side of each retina cross to the optic tract of the opposite side. The fibres from the temporal side of each retina pass back to the brain without decussation. Thus it will be seen that the right optic tract is made up of the fibres which supply the right side of each retina and the left optic tract the fibres of the left side of each retina (Fig. 16). The principal termination of the optic tracts is in the *cuneus* of the occipital lobe. A small bundle is sent to the nucleus of the third nerve.

LESSON V.

REFRACTION AND PHYSIOLOGY.

REFRACTION.

Refraction is the change which takes place in the direction of rays of light when they pass *obliquely* from one transparent medium into another of different density. Rays which pass into the second medium perpendicular to its surface are not deviated (*a a*, Fig. 17).

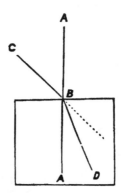

FIG. 17.—AA, perpendicular to surface between air and glass. C B D, ray bent toward perpendicular when passing from rarer medium air into denser medium glass. Reverse the direction and D B C is a ray bent from the perpendicular when passing from the denser medium glass into the rarer medium air.

All transparent solids and liquids are denser than air. They offer greater resistance to the transmission of light.

A ray of light passing from a rarer into a denser medium is bent toward the perpendicular. A ray of light passing from a denser into a rarer medium is bent from the perpendicular (Fig. 17). The degree of the deviation depends upon the difference in the density of the two media.

A *refracting prism* is any transparent body lying between two plane faces which are not parallel. A ray of light upon entering a prism is bent toward the perpendicular,

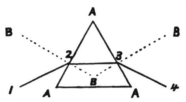

FIG. 18. — A A A, a prism; B B B, perpendiculars to sides of prism; 1, 2, 3, ray bent toward perpendicular when passing from air into glass; 2, 3, 4, ray bent from perpendicular when passing from glass into air.

upon emerging is bent from the perpendicular. A prism always bends rays toward its base (Fig. 18), and the image of an object seen through a prism is displaced toward its apex (Fig. 19).

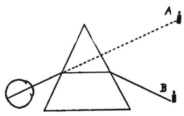

FIG. 19. — The image of the candle B, is displaced toward the apex of the prism and is seen at A.

Any transparent medium bounded by two curved surfaces, or one plane and the other curved, is a *lens*.

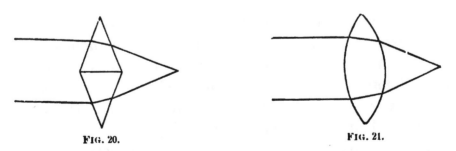

FIG. 20.   FIG. 21.

A *convex* lens may be regarded as a series of prisms with their bases directed toward the center (Fig 20). A convex lens converges parallel rays of light so as to bring them to a focus (Fig. 21). The distance from the optical center of a convex lens to the point where parallel rays are brought together is called its focal distance. Rays which diverge from a point corresponding with the focal distance of a convex lens are rendered parallel.

A *concave* lens may be regarded as a series of prisms with their bases directed from the center (Fig. 22). A concave lens diverges parallel rays of light (Fig. 23). If these rays be traced backwards they will come together at a point, the distance from which to the optical center of the lens is called its focal distance.

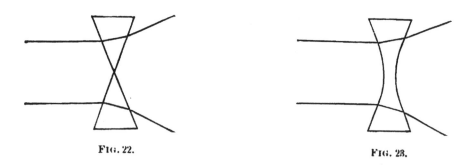

FIG. 22.   FIG. 23.

The strength of a lens or its ability to change the direction of rays depends upon the density of the material of which it is made and the degree of curvature of its surfaces.

The greater the strength of a lens the shorter is its focal distance. The term dioptre is used in numbering lenses. A lens whose focal distance is one metre is called a one dioptre lens, or 1.D. A lens of two metres focus has only one half the refractive power of a 1.D lens and is called a half dioptre lens, or 0.50 D. If the focal distance is one quarter of a metre it is a 4.D lens, etc.

Convex lenses are designated + (plus); concave lenses — (minus).

The average width of the pupil is 4 mm., and rays which enter it from a point 6 metres (20 feet) distant necessarily diverge very slightly. Therefore, rays from this distance and greater are arbitrarily considered parallel. When from a point under 6 metres, they are considered divergent.

In order that an eye may have distinct vision of an object, rays of light from that object must be brought to a focus on the retina. The cornea and crystalline lens act as convex lenses in bringing rays of light which enter the eye to a focus on the retina.

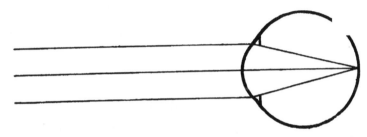

FIG. 24. — Parallel rays of light brought to a focus on the retina as in the emmétropic eye.

EMMETROPIA.

An eye, which in a state of rest brings parallel rays of light to a focus on its retina, has normal refraction and is called emmetropic.

ACCOMMODATION.

Rays from a near object are divergent, and in order for an emmetropic eye to have distinct vision of a near object it must increase its focal power, as it not only has to focus parallel rays, but has first to make the divergence parallel. This is accomplished by contracting the ciliary muscle. Contraction of the ciliary muscle relaxes the suspensory ligament and capsule of the lens. When the pressure of the capsule is relieved the lens becomes more convex by an inherent elasticity. Increase in its convexity increases its focusing power. This power the eye possesses of increasing its focal strength is called accommodation.

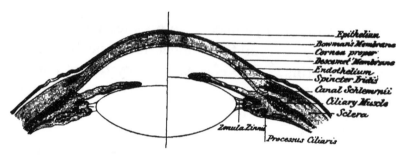

FIG. 25. — The left half represents the eye at rest, the right during accommodation. (Fick.)

PRESBYOPIA.

The elasticity of the crystalline lens diminishes gradually from childhood to old age. Under normal conditions this loss of elasticity is not felt until about the forty-fifth year, but at this period the power of accommodating is so lessened that convex glasses have to be resorted to for near vision. This physiological loss of accommodative power is called presbyopia. As accommodation diminishes the reading glass must be strengthened, necessitating a change about every two years.

HYPEROPIA.

If the focus of parallel rays is at an imaginary point behind the retina, the eye being at rest (*i. e.*, not accommodating), it is far-sighted or hyperopic. Hyperopia is due to shortness of the antero-posterior axis of the eyeball or to lack of sufficient focal strength in the cornea and lens. Since by accommodating the lens can increase its focal strength, hyperopic eyes accommodate constantly. Distant objects are seen plainly unless the 1y)ero)ia be very)ronounced. Near work is difficult and often painful.

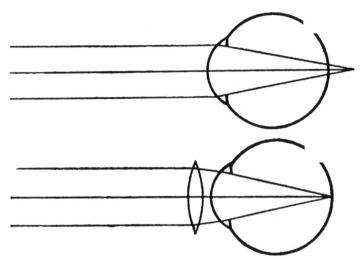

FIG. 26. — The upper figure shows parallel rays of light focused behind the retina as in hyperopia. The lower figure shows th · influence of a convex lens in bringing the focus to the retina.

We com)ensate for the lack of focal strengt1 and relieve the ciliary muscle of its strain by the use of convex lenses (Fig. 26).

LESSON VI.

REFRACTION AND PHYSIOLOGY (*Continued*).

MYOPIA.

If the focus of parallel rays is at a point in front of the retina, the eye being at rest, it is near-sighted or myopic. Myopia is due to too great length of the antero-posterior axis of the eyeball, or to too great focal strength of the cornea and lens. Since there is no way of decreasing the focal strength of the lens, no effort on the part of a myope

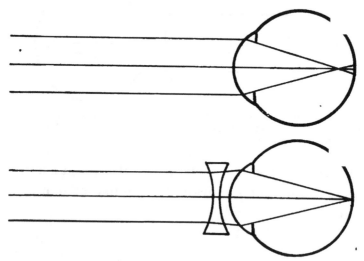

FIG. 27.—The upper figure shows parallel rays of light focused in front of the retina as in myopia. The lower figure shows the influence of a concave lens in moving the focus back to the retina.

can overcome his defect. Distant objects are seen poorly, and, if the myopia is pronounced, are not seen at all. Myopia is corrected by the use of concave lenses (Fig. 27).

In hyperopia the effort of accommodation necessitates the constant exercise of the circular fibres of the ciliary muscle, and we find in hyperopic eyes that the circular fibres are increased in size and number as in figure 28.

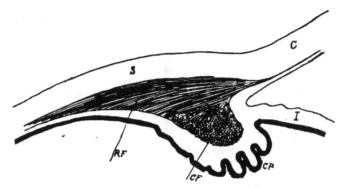

FIG. 28.—Ciliary muscle of a hyperopic eye. R F, radiating fibres; C F, circular fibres.

Accommodation would make the vision of a myopic eye worse, and we find in these eyes that the circular fibres of the ciliary muscle are small in size and number, as in figure 29.

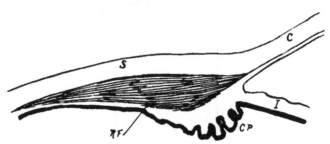

FIG. 29.—Ciliary muscle of a myopic eye.

ASTIGMATISM.

In emmetropia, hyperopia and myopia, the curvature of the cornea is the same in every meridian, and its refracting power is the same through every part, vertical, horizontal and oblique. All rays that enter these eyes are brought to a common focus. Sometimes the cornea has meridians of different curvature producing greater refraction in some meridians than in others. Such a condition constitutes astigmatism. In astigmatism the rays passing tirough the meridian of greatest refraction reach their focus nearest the cornea, wiile tiose passing tirougi the least refracting meridian come to a focus fartiest back.

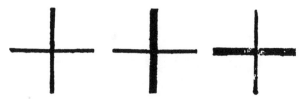

FIG. 30.—Cross lines as seen by an emmetropic eye and by two astigmatic eyes. (Juler.)

The meridians of iigiest and lowest refracting power are at rigit angles to eaci otier and are called the *principal meridians*. Astigmatism is sometimes due to unequal curvature of the meridians of the crystalline lens or to an oblique position of the lens witi regard to rays entering

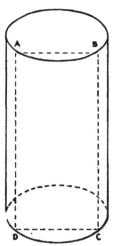

FIG. 31.—A, B, C, D is a section of a cylinder cut parallel to its axis.

the pupil. To correct astigmatism we employ a lens which is a section of a cylinder parallel to its axis (Fig. 31). Rays passing tirougi the axis of a cylindrical lens are not refracted. Rays passing tirougi the meridian wiich is perpendicular to the axis undergo the maximum refraction. The refracting value of any meridian lying between these two principal meridians depends upon its proximity to the region of no refraction (the axis), or to the region of maximum refraction (Fig. 32).

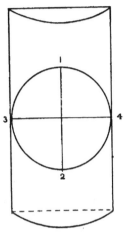

FIG. 32.— A lens cut from a section of a cylinder. The meridian 1, 2, is parallel to the axis of the cylinder, it has no curvature and no refracting power. The meridian, 3, 4, being thicker at the middle than at the ends, is convex; it will bring parallel rays of light to a focus.

CONVERGENCE.

When an eye is directed toward an object so that the image of the thing looked at falls upon the fovea centralis, the eye is said to fix that object. Normally both eyes fix the same object, and in order to do this when it is brought near to the face, both eyes have to turn inward; the nearer the object the more the eyes turn in. The turning in of the eyes necessary to fix near objects is called convergence.

FIELD OF VISION.

When the eye is fixed on an object, other things besides the one looked at are visible. Those nearest the one fixed are most distinct and the greater the distance of an object from the one fixed, the less distinctly is it seen. That area in which objects are visible, the eye being fixed, is the field of vision. It will be seen from Fig. 33 that the nasal

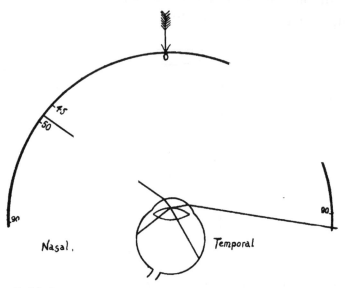

FIG. 33.—Field of vision of a right eye. The arrow at o being fixed (looked at) all objects on the temporal side within the area described by about 95 degrees of a circle are visible; all objects on the nasal side within about 48 degrees are visible. The nasal side of the field is restricted by the bridge of the nose.

field of each eye extends to about 48 degrees from the object looked at, therefore if both eyes look at the same object there is an overlapping of the two fields or an area that is common to both eyes. This area which extends to about 48 degrees on each side of the object is called the binocular field of vision.

COLOR PERCEPTION.

A ray of sunlight passed through a prism and projected upon a screen forms a band of colors ranging from red to violet. The red is toward the apex and the violet toward the base of the prism. Between the red and violet there are gradations of orange, yellow, green and blue. The wave lengths of these colored rays gradually decrease from the red rays which are .000760 mm., to the violet, which are .000397 mm. The greater the wave length of a ray of light, the less it is deviated by passing through a medium of different density, hence the power of a prism to separate a ray of white light into its elements. The six colors of the solar spectrum, red, orange, yellow, green, blue and violet, are called *simple colors* because it is found by passing any one of them through a prism that no further disintegration takes place (Fig. 34). Red, green and violet can be mixed to produce any of the other colors, but as no combination can produce either of these three they are called the *primary colors*.

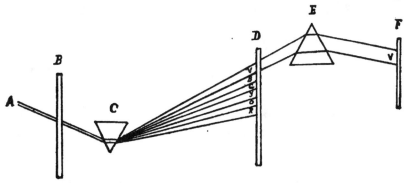

FIG. 34.— B is a screen which intercepts all rays of light except the ray A. The prism C separates the ray A into the simple colors, red, orange, yellow, green, blue and violet, which are thrown on the screen D. The violet rays, if passed through the screen D, and prism E, would show on the screen F, as violet; no further disintegration taking place.

Many theories have been offered to explain the phenomenon of color perception, but none has yet supplanted the Young-Helmholtz. This is that we have three primary color perceptions corresponding to the three primary colors of nature, and that there are red perceptive fibres, green perceptive fibres and violet perceptive fibres in our retinas. These different nerve fibres are stimulated by light waves of different lengths. Equal stimulation of all three produces the sensation of white, and just as all the colors in

nature can be produced by mixing the spectrum red, green
and violet, so can every color sensation be produced by
stimulation of the red, green and violet perceptive fibres in
varying proportions. The absence or impairment of one
or more of the primary perceptions constitutes *color-
blindness;* the characteristic of the defect depending upon

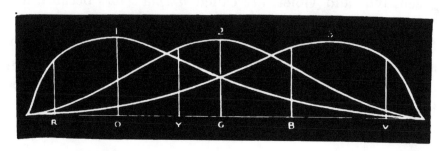

FIG. 35. — A diagram of color perception. 1, Red; 2, Green; 3, Violet. The height
of the curve from the base line indicates the proportions in which the primary
colors are mixed to produce the simple colors of the spectrum, red, orange, yellow
green, blue and violet.

which element is missing or impaired. The condition is
congenital, does not disturb vision, is not dependent upon
any demonstrable pathological lesion, is irremediable and is
often hereditary. There are other forms of color-blind-
ness depending upon diseases of the retina and optic nerve,
which will be described in connection with those diseases-

LESSON VII.

DISEASES OF THE OCULAR MUSCLES.

STRABISMUS.

Normally, both eyes fix the same object. The image of the object looked at falls upon the fovea centralis of both eyes. This is accomplished by the co-ordination and association of movement of the six external ocular muscles of

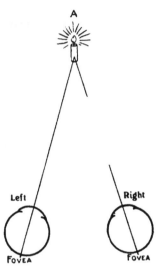

FIG. 36. — The two eyes in a state of muscular equilibrium. The image of the candle A falls upon the fovea centralis of each eye.

each eye. In looking up, down, right or left, the eyes move together and binocular or single vision results, because the images of objects in the field of vision fall upon *identical parts* of each retina, the upper half of the right retina corresponding to the upper half of the left, the right or temporal side of the right retina to the right or nasal side of the left, etc. In this **normal state the eyes are said** to be balanced or **in equilib**

If this association of movement is disturbed, so that the image of an object falls upon the fovea centralis of one eye and not upon the fovea of the other, we have strabismus, or squint. The eye which receives the image of the object looked at upon its fovea is called the *fixing eye;* the other is called the squinting, or *deviating eye.* The deviation may be in any direction, depending upon which muscle or set of muscles is affected.

Strabismus is either paralytic or concomitant.

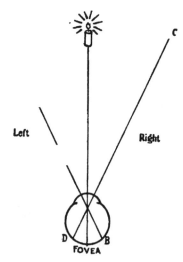

FIG. 37.—The eye is fixed on the candle. Objects in the right field at C are perceived by the left side of the retina at D. Objects at A are perceived by the right retina at B.

PARALYTIC STRABISMUS

Is produced by loss of power in one or more of the ocular muscles. This loss of power may be total (paralysis) or partial (paresis), the latter being by far the more frequent.

Symptoms. — 1. **Movement of the eye** in the direction of the action of the affected muscle is limited or lost. If an external rectus is paretic its antagonist, the internal rectus, will pull the eye inward. The deviation of the afflicted

eye, the sound eye fixing, is called the *primary deviation*.
If the sound eye be covered by a card and the paretic eye
fixes the object, it will be seen by looking behind the card
that the sound eye has now deviated in a direction opposite
to the primary deviation, and that the deviation is greater.
This is called the *secondary deviation*. In paralytic strabismus the secondary deviation is always greater than the
primary, because the same amount of nervous impulse necessary to produce a given result in the weakened muscle is
also conveyed to its sound associate and results in its over-
action.

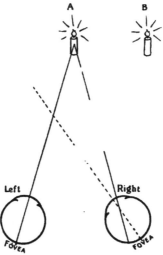

FIG. 38.—Convergent strabismus of the right eye. The image of the candle A,
falls on the retina at the inner side of the fovea and is seen at B. Homonymous
diplopia. A, true image. B, false image.

2. **Diplopia** or double vision results because the muscular imbalance or lack of equilibrium prevents images of
objects in the field of vision from falling upon the identical parts of each retina. If an external rectus is paralyzed
the anterior pole turns in, the posterior pole out. The
image of the object fixed by the sound eye falls upon the
retina of the diseased eye, to the inner side of the fovea
centralis and is projected to the temporal side of its field.

This is due to the fact that the patient is in the habit of
locating objects in the temporal field which are perceived
by the nasal side of the retina (Fig. 37) and he does not
take into consideration the deviation of his eye. If it
is an internal rectus that is weakened the eye turns outward and the image of the object fixed by the sound eye
falls on the retina of the diseased eye to the outer side of
its fovea and is projected to the nasal side of the field.

Thus it will be seen when the strabismus is convergent
the image of the right eye is on the right side, the image
of the left eye on the left side. This is called *homonymous diplopia* (Fig. 38).

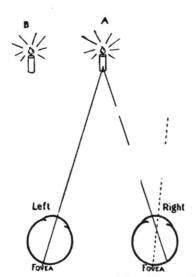

FIG. 39. — Divergent strabismus of the right eye. The image of the candle A.
falls on the retina at the outer side of the fovea and is seen at B. Heteronymous
diplopia. A. true image. B. false image.

When the strabismus is divergent the image of the right
eye is to the left, the image of the left eye to the right.
This is called crossed or *heteronymous diplopia* (Fig. 39).
In vertical strabismus the lower image belongs to the eye
turned up, the upper image to the eye directed downward.

3. Inaccuracy in the determination of the position of objects in that part of the field toward which the affected muscle normally directs the eye is observed in paralytic strabismus. In looking toward an object on our right side, we determine by experience its distance to the right by the amount of innervation necessary to direct the visual axes toward it. If the right external rectus muscle is paretic an unusual amount of energy is necessary to fix the object and it will seem farther toward the right side than it really is.

4. Vertigo, nausea and headache are troublesome features of paralytic strabismus. The vertigo is produced by diplopia and by the inability to properly locate objects in part of the field of vision.

5. A peculiar carriage of the head will be observed. It will be turned in such a way as to overcome the diplopia by excluding the paretic muscle. If the right external rectus muscle is weakened the face will be turned toward the right side, which is equivalent to directing the gaze to the left, in which act the paretic muscle would have to take no part.

Cause.—The cause may be found in the brain, the nerve-trunk, or in the muscle itself. It is due to syphilis in about half of all cases and in the other half to exposure to cold, rheumatism, diphtheria, tabes dorsalis, diabetes, poisons, tumors, meningitis, aneurism, periostitis, hemorrhage, wounds, fractures, and hysteria.

Treatment.—The subjective symptoms can be relieved at once by covering the diseased eye. If the patient wears glasses, a ground glass on that side is effective. Treatment of paralytic strabismus must depend upon the cause. When due to syphilis or rheumatism, the remedies appropriate to these conditions are indicated. When the result of debilitating causes, such as diphtheria, chronic poisoning, etc., give general tonics including strychnin. A weak current of electricity may be tried. the positive pole being placed over the affected muscle, the negative pole on the back of the neck. When the deviation is slight and has become fixed, relief is often afforded by wearing prisms. In selected cases operative treatment, tenotomy or advancement, may be helpful.

LESSON VIII.

DISEASES OF THE OCULAR MUSCLES (*Continued*).

CONCOMITANT STRABISMUS.

Symptoms. — There is an absence of the normal association of movement of the ocular muscles without loss of their power. The muscles have their normal strength, but they do not work together so that each eye will fix the same object at the same time. The primary and secondary deviations are equal. The deviation may be *monolateral* or *alternating;* if the latter, vision in each eye will probably be the same. It is a condition which usually manifests itself early in life, the average age being about three years. Diplopia is rare in concomitant strabismus; the squinting eye is often so amblyopic as not to perceive the false image, and if it has good vision, concomitant squint arises so early in life that there is developed, with the growth of the child, a power of the mind to exclude the false image.

Cause. — There is more to discover relative to the cause of concomitant strabismus than has yet been revealed, but the following may be given as etiological factors : —

1. **Hyperopia** exists in three-fourths of all cases of internal, concomitant strabismus. Convergence and accommodation are associated actions, and in hyperopia there is excessive accommodation and the associated convergence sometimes amounts to internal strabismus. Relief of the hyperopia by convex glasses will at times straighten these eyes. But that hyperopia is not a prime factor in the production of strabismus is proven by the fact that, in the majority of cases, the correction of the hyperopia by glasses has no effect on the strabismus, and also that there are so many

cases of high degree of hyperopia in which there is no strabismus.

2. **Myopia** is associated with divergent strabismus and the explanation is that the convergence necessary to focus at the far point of a myopic eye, which is very close to the face, puts too great a strain on the internal rectus muscles, one of them gives up and divergence results. The exception to this rule is proven by the fact that only a very small proportion of the cases of myopia diverge.

3. **Amblyopia** or poor vision in the squinting eye is found in many cases of strabismus (72 per cent, Nagel) and the weight of authority is in favor of the view that the amblyopia is congenital and is the cause of the strabismus, the stimulation to binocular vision not being present. However, a respectable minority claim the amblyopia to be the effect of non-use of the squinting eye and not the cause of the strabismus. But that congenital amblyopia is only a factor in the production of squint is proven by the absence of squint in the majority of amblyopic eyes.

4. **Unusual development of a single ocular muscle** is another possible element in the production of concomitant strabismus, the internal rectus being often unnaturally strong in internal strabismus and the same is true of the external rectus when the deviation is outward.

Treatment. — Rarely concomitant strabismus disappears without medical aid. Sometimes it is entirely removed by wearing the glass which corrects the refractive error, consequently these eyes should be tested and the proper glasses ordered as soon as the child is old enough to wear them. It is also good practice to cover the fixing eye with a bandage for a part of each day to compel the use of the deviating eye.

The treatment for the remaining cases is operative, tenotomy of the over-active muscle or advancement of its antagonist. Operations for strabismus should not be performed before twelve or fifteen years of age, except in rare cases, owing to the tendency to development of over-effect with the growth of the child.

INSUFFICIENCY OF THE OCULAR MUSCLES OR LATENT SQUINT.

This condition differs from strabismus only in degree, the tendency to deviation being overcome by the desire for binocular vision. It may be concomitant or paretic. There is lack of balance of the ocular muscles but parallelism of the visual lines is maintained. The effort to maintain this parallelism and secure binocular vision generally results in *asthenopia*, which may be manifested by pain over the insertion of the weak muscle, blurred vision, inability to do close or protracted work, photophobia, subacute congestion of the conjunctiva, headache, vertigo and other neuroses

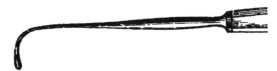

FIG. 40.—Strabismus hook used to pick up the ocular muscle in performing tenotomy.

Treatment.—The treatment of this condition is difficult and belongs to the oculist. Careful correction of any refractive error is of first importance. The constitution should be appropriately treated and use of the eyes regulated. In some cases wearing prisms gives relief. There are methods of exercising the weak muscle which may restore the necessary power. As a last resort operative measures may be adopted, which consist in partial tenotomy of the over-active muscle or advancement of the weak one.

NYSTAGMUS.

This condition is characterized by rapid, involuntary oscillation of the eyeballs, generally in the lateral direction. It may be congenital or acquired and nearly always affects both eyes. If acquired, the patient will, at first, complain of the movement of objects looked at.

Cause. — Defective development of the eyes, albinism, bad vision from corneal and lenticular opacities, blindness and protracted use of the eyes in an abnormal position, it being common with miners, who work with their eyes directed obliquely upward. It is also due to brain lesions of central origin, ataxia and tumors of the cerebellum.

Treatment. — Improve vision by all possible means; if there is any refractive error put on the correcting glass, if there is a central corneal scar make a false pupil. In case of strabismus do a tenotomy, and if the occupation is at fault change it at once. The great majority of cases of nystagmus get little or no relief.

LESSON IX.

DISEASES OF THE LIDS.

BLEPHARITIS.

This is an inflammation of the lid border characterized by the following symptoms given in the order of their severity. 1. Hyperemia, itching and slight swelling. 2. Seborrhea or hypersecretion of the sebaceous glands. The dried sebum forms yellow crusts on the border of the lid. 3. Ulceration at the root of the lashes. 4. Thickening of the edge of the lid. 5. Falling of eyelashes with atrophy of their follicles. 6. Ectropium with eversion of the lacrymal puncta and resulting epiphora.

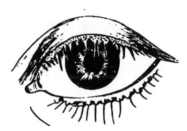

FIG. 41.—Blepharitis, eyelashes matted into bundles by the secretion along lid borders.

Cause. — It is sometimes eczematous in nature and is most frequently found in the fair-skinned, the strumous and the badly nourished. Chronic conjunctivitis and lacrymal obstruction are causative. Some error of refraction may be present.

Treatment. — Correct the refractive error. Protect eyes from the irritation of dust, smoke, etc. Treat the constitution with cod liver oil, iron and arsenic if struma or debility are present. If there are ulcers around the cilia pull

out the lashes so affected and touch the ulcers with nitrate
of silver stick. Rub into the edge of lids, once a day,
an ointment of the yellow oxid of mercury, gr. $\frac{1}{2}$ to
vaseline 3i. or an ointment of ammoniated mercury, gr. $\frac{1}{3}$
to 3j. Before applying the ointment all secretion should be
cleansed from the lid border. Eight grains of biborate of
soda to one ounce of warm water will be found useful in
removing the crusts. If there is lacrymal obstruction it
must receive appropriate attention. In the chronic stage
of blepharitis stimulating tar ointments are recommended
but in the majority of cases mild and soothing measures
will be the most efficacious.

HORDEOLUM.

A stye is an acute inflammation of a sebaceous gland at
the lid border. It is usually, in appearance and symptoms,
a small boil but sometimes produces general edema of the
lid with chemosis of the conjunctiva.

Cause. — Error of refraction, general debility, possibly
germ infection.

Treatment. — Use hot applications to bring the inflammation to a focus, then open. Correct the constitutional condition if debility exists. Correct refractive errors and remove any source of local irritation. Sulfid of calcium,
$\frac{1}{2}$ grain twice a day or dilute sulfuric acid ten drops after
each meal may be given.

CHALAZION.

This small tumor of the lid is due to a chronic inflammation of a Meibomian gland. Its development is gradual
and usually without any symptoms which annoy the patient.
The inflammatory process causes proliferation of the epithelial lining of the gland and cell infiltration of the surrounding tissue. This inflamed area develops into a granula-

tion mass surrounded by a thin connective tissue capsule. The granuloma tends to break down in the center, forming a liquid, which may become purulent. Rarely the mass becomes fibrous and solid.

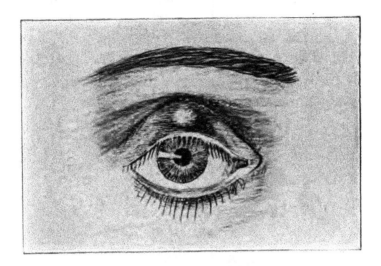

FIG. 42. — Chalazion of upper lid.

Treatment. — The contents may escape and the tumor disappear spontaneously, but more frequently it is necessary to cut down upon it and if it is soft, curette it, if hard and fibrous, dissect it out. The incision may be made

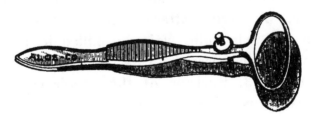

FIG. 43. — Clamp used in removing small tumors from the lids.

through the skin if destruction of the tarsus has rendered it subcutaneous, otherwise it is better to evacuate it through the conjunctiva.

TRICHIASIS.

Wild hairs, misplaced or misdirected eyelashes rubbing the globe, produce great pain and blepharospasm and may cause ulceration and subsequent opacity of the cornea.

Cause. — If the trichiasis is partial it may be congenital or may be due to the cicatricial contraction following styes, blepharitis ulcerosa, traumatism, etc. If there is a complete trichiasis it is usually associated with entropium and is, as a rule, the result of trachoma.

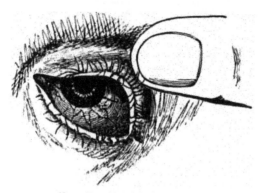

FIG. 44. — Trichiasis. (Wells.)

Treatment. — 1. Epilation or pulling out of the offending hairs is only of temporary benefit, as they grow in again. 2. Electrolysis, introduced by Michel of St. Louis, is valuable. A needle attached to the negative pole is passed to the hair bulb, which is killed by a current of about five milliamperes. This procedure is exceedingly painful. 3. Excision of the misplaced hairs with their bulbs is useful when they are few in number and close together. 4. If the wild hairs are isolated their direction can be changed by passing a needle, threaded with a loop, through the lid in the direction you wish the hair to take, then catching the hair in the loop and drawing it through the tissues as you pull the thread through.

5. When the trichiasis is total and the lid border is turned inward, one of the operations for entropium should be done.

ENTROPIUM AND ECTROPIUM.

Entropium is a turning in of the lid. Ectropium is a turning out of the lid.

1. We have spasmodic entropium and spasmodic ectropium.

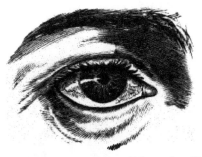

FIG. 45.—Entropium of the lower lid.   (After Mackenzie.)

Spasmodic contraction of the fibres of the orbicularis near the lid border in conjunction with a relaxed and flabby skin and a deep set eyeball causes the lid border to turn inward producing spasmodic entropium, which is nearly always found in the aged. This condition occurs almost without exception in the lower lid. Spasmodic contraction of the fibres of the orbicularis farthest from the lid border, in conjunction with a tense skin, congested and thickened conjunctiva or a prominent eyeball, causes the lid border to turn outward producing spasmodic ectropium, which is nearly always found in children and young people.

2. We have cicatricial entropium and cicatricial ectropium.

Trachoma, some forms of conjunctivitis and wounds may produce cicatricial contraction of the conjunctiva lining the

lid wiici turns the edge of the lid inward, causing entro-
)ium.

Burns, wounds, ulcers, caries of the orbital border and
otier causes may)roduce cicatricial contraction of the skin
of the lid, wiici turns the edge of the lid outward, causing
ectro)ium.

We iave, in addition to the above conditions, a)aralytic
ectro)ium due to paralysis of the orbicularis muscle. The
lower lid falls outward and away from the globe by its own
weigit. The lower lid is the only one affected by)aralytic
ectro)ium.

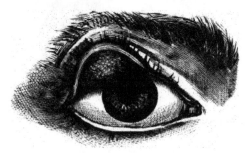

FIG. 46.—Ectropium of upper lid. (After Lawson.)

The treatment is almost always o)erative. S)asmodic
entro)ium can be tem)orarily relieved by)ainting the skin
over the inferior orbital margin witi collodium, contraction
of wiici everts the lid border.

DISEASES OF THE LIDS (*Continued*).

BLEPHAROSPASM.

Spasm of the orbicularis appears under a variety of forms: 1. Abnormal frequency of winking or nictitation may be an unconscious habit which sometimes lasts a lifetime. 2. A similar manifestation is seen in children, due to chronic conjunctivitis, but it may be the beginning of a general chorea. 3. In hysteria there is sometimes pronounced blepharospasm, which may be tonic or clonic. 4. In old age a tonic blepharospasm, which resists all treatment, may occur (Fuchs). 5. A reflex spasm of the orbicularis may be due to trichiasis, corneal and conjunctival diseases, foreign bodies, errors of refraction, and to any condition which can cause photophobia. Treatment is to remove the cause. 6. There is a clonic form of blepharospasm corresponding with tic douloureux, which is very painful. At given intervals the cramp seizes the orbicularis and other muscles of one side of the face, causing distortion and great pain. The paroxysm passes off in about a minute, to be repeated again after an interval varying in length in different cases. I have seen it return four or six times in an hour. The cause is some nerve or brain lesion, and treatment is very ineffectual. Iodid and bromid of potassium have each been beneficial. If any peripheral, exciting cause can be discovered, it should be removed.

LAGOPHTHALMIA.

Lagophthalmia is an inability to close the lids. Constant exposure of the globe causes conjunctivitis, ulceration of the cornea, and an overflow of tears, due to the mal-position of the punctum. The evils of lagophthalmia are lessened by the tendency of the cornea to turn upward under the lid when an effort to close the palpebral fissure is made. This also occurs in sleep.

Cause. — 1. Protrusion of the eyeball as in ex-ophthalmic goitre or orbital tumors. 2. Large anterior staphyloma. 3. Congenital shortening of the lids. 4. Loss of lid tissue from lupus, burns, etc. 5. Ectropium. 6. Paralysis of the seventh nerve. The course of this nerve is long and devious, and it passes through numerous tissues, which exposes it to accident or disease.

Treatment. — The treatment consists in removing the cause, meanwhile protecting the cornea from irritation by covering the eye with a bandage or holding the lids together with adhesive plaster. In the erect position, the force of gravity will help to draw the lid down over the cornea. In some cases tarsorrhaphy is necessary. This consists in shortening the palpebral fissure by uniting the edges of the lids.

PTOSIS.

Ptosis is a complete or partial drooping of the upper lid. If congenital, it is frequently bilateral; when acquired it is generally unilateral.

Cause. — The causes of congenital ptosis are: 1. Deficient development or absence of the levator palpebrae superioris muscle. 2. Injury inflicted by the forceps in difficult delivery. 3. Defective attachment of the skin to the underlying tissues, producing that form called ptosis adiposa, in which the skin falls over the lid border like a pouch.

The causes of acquired ptosis are: 1. Injury to the levator muscle. 2. Paralysis of the third nerve, usually from syphilis (Fig. 47). 3. Thickening of the lids by new growths, trachoma, etc. 4. Hysteria.

Treatment. — Attack the cause when it can be located. The congenital forms require operations. In paralysis use anti-syphilitic and anti-rheumatic measures. Electricity, one pole back of the ear and the other over the lid, may be tried.

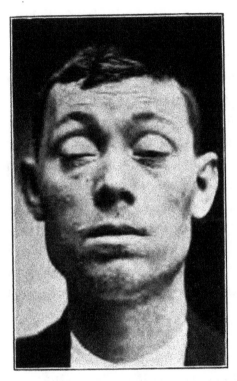

Fig. 47. — Acquired ptosis of syphilitic origin. The effort to raise the lids by elevating the eyebrows is shown.

ECZEMA.

Eczema of the lids is most frequently met with in children who have phlyctenular ophthalmia, and in adults with an irritating discharge from the eye. The symptoms and treatment are the same as of eczema in other parts. In an acute case treatment should be mild and soothing, when chronic it can be more stimulating. Dust with starch powder or aristol. Apply oxid of zinc ointment to whici carbolic acid, 5 grains to the ounce, may be added. Yellow oxid of mercury ointment is useful, as is also painting with nitrate of silver solution, 10 to 20 grains to the ounce.

HERPES ZOSTER OPHTHALMICUS.

This term is applied to shingles following the course of the first and second divisions of the fifth nerve. It is characterized by redness and swelling of the skin and the formation of vesicles on the forehead, eyelids and nose. The disease is very painful and is a menace to sight if the vesicular eruption appears on the cornea. A severe neuralgia generally precedes the attack and may persist for a long time after it. The cause of the disease is an inflammation of the fifth nerve of an obscure character. Treatment is unsatisfactory. The vesicles should not be ruptured and when they dry forming crusts, the latter should remain undisturbed. Picking off the crusts deepens the subsequent scars. Anodynes may be required. Internally salicylic acid and quinin have both been recommended.

PHTHIRIASIS.

Crab lice may get into the eyelashes and give rise to excessive itching; the consequent rubbing and scratching of the lids sets up a mild inflammation which may be mistaken for blepharitis. The lice and their eggs may be seen on the cilia. Treatment is to rub the lid border and lashes thoroughly with mercurial ointment every night until the parasites are killed.

ECCHYMOSIS OF THE LIDS.

A " black eye " is the result of any cause which ruptures a blood vessel of the sub-cutaneous tissue of the lid. It is most frequently due to a blow. Time is the only cure. A bandage, cold a)) lications immediately after the accident, arnica or lead and o) ium wash will assist.

Erysi) elas, abscess, sy)) ilitic sore, ulcer, nevus, epithelioma, sarcoma, lu) us and molluscum contagiosum are all diseases t) at may be found on the lids but t) eir descriptions belong more properly to a work less limited in character.

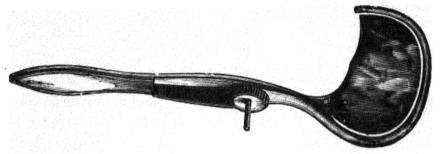

FIG. 48.—Clamp used to prevent hemorrhage and steady the part in lid operations

THE LACRYMAL APPARATUS AND ORBITS.

DISEASES OF THE LACRYMAL APPARATUS.

The lacrymal system is divided into a *secretory* part, the glands, and an *excretory* or drainage part, the puncta, canaliculi, sac and duct. Normally the lacrymal secretion is about balanced by evaporation. In acute diseases of the eye and under the influence of certain emotions there is pronounced hypersecretion of tears, or lacrymation, and the excretory apparatus being unable to carry them off, they overflow on to the cheeks. In chronic eye diseases there is a slight hypersecretion of tears and if the drainage apparatus be normal they will be carried off through the natural channels. If the drainage is impaired, by eversion or occlusion of the puncta, plugging or stricture of the canaliculi or stricture of the duct, etc., the fluid cannot find a natural outlet and the eye is bathed in tears which drip over the edge of the lid. This condition is called *epiphora*.

DISEASES OF THE LACRYMAL GLAND.

1. **Inflammation** of the lacrymal gland occurs very rarely. There would be the usual symptoms of inflammation which might result in suppuration of the surrounding connective tissue or recover without it. There is often difficulty in excluding orbital cellulitis, phlegmon of the lid and periostitis. Treatment consists of hot bichlorid fomentation, anodynes and evacuation of the pus if formed.

2. **Dislocation** of the lacrymal gland appears as a movable tumor under the ocular conjunctiva at the upper

and outer part of the globe. Treatment does not avail. Extirpation may be resorted to.

3. **Tumors** of numerous varieties may develop in the lacrymal gland. Hypertrophy and atrophy have been observed.

4. **Fistula** of the gland is generally the result of an abscess or injury. A connection with the conjunctival sac should be established, then the cutaneous opening is easily closed by cauterization.

5. **Dacryops** is the term applied to a bluish, translucent, soft tumor which appears in the upper and outer conjunctival fornix. It is caused by the occlusion of one or more of the ducts which convey the lacrymal fluid from the gland into the conjunctival sac. As the tumor is a distended duct filled with tears it will collapse if punctured and the treatment consists in establishing a permanent opening.

ANOMALIES OF THE PUNCTA AND CANALICULI.

1. **Eversion,** or falling of the lower punctum away from the eyeball, may be due to ectropium, chronic conjunctivitis or blepharitis marginalis.

2. **Obliteration** of a punctum or canaliculus may be congenital or may result from traumatism or chronic inflammation.

3. **Obstruction** of a canaliculus by a foreign body sometimes occurs.

CHRONIC DACRYOCYSTITIS.

This is a catarrhal inflammation of the sac and duct. *Stricture of the duct* will also be included under this head as these conditions merge into each other and are more or less interdependent.

Symptoms. — A slight catarrhal inflammation of the mucous membrane of the sac and duct, creates a muco-purulent discharge, some of which passes backward through the puncta and produces a mild conjunctivitis and epiphora. This slight attack may disappear without treatment, or upon the instillation of some mild antiseptic collyrium and the appropriate attention to the nose. If the inflammation is more severe, the swelling of the mucous membrane will produce an occlusion of the duct and a consequent accumulation of the contents of the sac. The muco-purulent contents will become purulent, and will escape through the puncta and excite a conjunctivitis. With this conjunctivitis there will be hypersecretion of tears and epiphora.

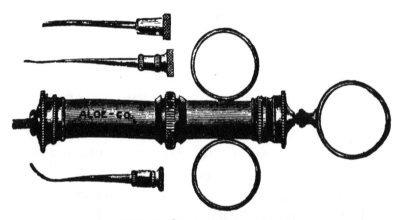

FIG. 49. — Anel's syringe, used to wash out the lachrymal sac and duct.

The accumulation of fluid in the sac produces a tumefaction which will disappear upon pressure, as the fluid is forced back through the puncta or through the stricture into the nose. The stenosis of the duct may be complete. The purulent contents of the distended sac are extremely toxic and will almost surely infect a wound of the cornea, will often light up an active inflammation of the connective tissue surrounding the sac (acute dacryocystitis), and may, if of long standing, produce caries of adjacent bone.

Cause. — Dacryocystitis may be started by any of the numerous causes of inflammation of mucous membrane, such as temperature changes and infection. Stricture of the duct will cause a dacryocystitis, and stricture may be due to morbid conditions of the nasal cavities, traumatism, asymetry of the face, deflected septum, periostitis or syphilis. The prognosis in chronic cases is bad. If cured they require months of treatment, and too often patients have not time or inclination to resort to the needed measures.

Treatment. — Teach patients to keep the sac empty by pressure. See that the nasal cavities are kept clean by washing them out with Dobell's solution. The mildest form is sometimes benefited by dropping into the eye, three times a day, a 1 to 2000 solution of blue pyoktanin. Wash out the sac with a 1 to 5000 solution of bichlorid of mercury every other day. If the discharge is purulent, inject into the sac a small quantity of a solution of nitrate of silver (gr. 2 to the ounce) or protargol (5 to 20 per cent), after having cleaned it out by washing with bichlorid of mercury or boracic acid solutions. If there be a stricture of the duct slit a canaliculus (upper preferred) and dilate the stricture with probes.

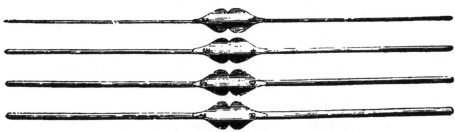

FIG. 50. — Bowman's probes for dilating the nasal duct.

ACUTE DACRYOCYSTITIS.

Symptoms. — In the course of a chronic dacryocystitis, a severe inflammation may suddenly develop in the region of the sac. There will be redness and swelling which will extend to the lids and conjunctiva. Pain will be very severe and there may be some fever. Pus will form and the skin over the abscess become thin. Unless opened the skin will break, emptying the contents of the abscess and establishing a *lacrymal fistula*. As soon as the pus is evacuated the symptoms rapidly subside, to recur as soon as the fistula is allowed to close.

Cause. — A lesion of the mucous membrane of a sac affected by chronic dacryocystitis, allows its toxic contents to infect the surrounding sub-mucous tissue and the active phlegmonous inflammation follows.

Treatment. — Evacuate the pus by slitting up a canaliculus if possible, if not open through the skin over the sac. Keep the incision open by gauze drainage until the abscess can be cleansed through a canaliculus and then treat as a chronic dacryocystitis.

DISEASES OF THE ORBITS.

From the position, structure and contents of the orbit we can readily conceive of some of the diseases which afflict it. We may have fractures of the bony walls; laceration of the soft parts by foreign bodies; emphysema caused by the escape of air from the lacrymal sac, the etmoid cells or frontal sinuses; profuse hemorrhage from injury or straining; periostitis from injury, or secondary to other inflammation, etc. These are surgical conditions and can be diagnosed and treated on the lines of general surgery. There are two symptoms so constantly attendant upon orbital disease as to make them worthy of special mention.

1. Proptosis or exophthalmos.
2. Limitation of movement of the eyeball.

Associated with these salient symptoms are injection and chemosis of the conjunctiva, redness, swelling and edema of the lids and severe pain, most noticeable when the patient attempts to move the globe, or the surgeon presses it backward into the orbit.

ORBITAL CELLULITIS.

This is an inflammation of the cellular tissue of the orbit.

Symptoms.— Proptosis with diplopia, pain, limitation of movement of the ball, injection and chemosis of the conjunctiva and swelling and redness of the lids. As the severity of this disease varies greatly in different cases, we shall expect variation in the degree of manifestations of all symptoms. In the severe forms there will be chills with fever, and may be loss of vision due to pressure upon the optic nerve or disturbance of the intra-ocular circulation. There may be ulceration of the cornea and possibly suppuration of the whole eyeball. The inflammation has been known to extend to the meninges of the brain.

Cause. — The causes are such as produce cellulitis in other locations and are numerous. Special mention may be made of the severe form due to erysipelas, and also to the fact that it may arise by metastasis in all pyemic conditions, especially puerperal septicemia.

Treatment. — Support with tonics, especially quinin and iron. Relieve pain by anodynes. Apply hot fomentation, and as soon as the abscess can be located or any sign of fluctuation appears, open and treat antiseptically.

TUMORS OF THE ORBIT

The orbit contains many different tissues, consequently a great variety of tumors may develop in this locality.

Exophthalmos and limitation of movement of the ball, without the usual manifestation of inflammation, are the most pronounced symptoms. Removal of the tumor is the treatment; without the ball if the nature and extent of the growth will admit, with it if necessary.

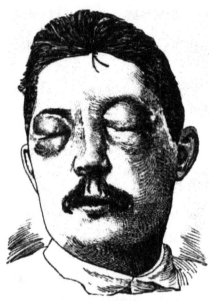

FIG. 51. — Double orbital cellulitis, the result of erysipelas. (De Schweinitz.)

Exophthalmos with congestion of the vessels of the conjunctiva and lid, pain, noises in the head, pulsation of the eyeball and a bruit heard over the orbital region are the symptoms of *pulsating exophthalmos*. It is generally due to an aneurism caused by a traumatic rupture of the carotid into the cavernous sinus. In rare instances it is due to an aneurism of the ophthalmic artery. Ligation or compression of the common carotid is the usual treatment. In cases caused by a diseased condition, which can be definitely located in the orbit, resection of the orbital wall and ligation of the ophthalmic vein has been advised.

LESSON XII.

DISEASES OF THE CONJUNCTIVA.

CATARRHAL CONJUNCTIVITIS.

This is the most frequent disease of the eye. It usually attacks both eyes, varies greatly in severity and duration, and tends to spontaneous recovery, rarely lasting over two weeks. *Hyperemia* of the conjunctiva is generally given as a separate disease but practically differs from simple catarrhal conjunctivitis only in degree, being milder.

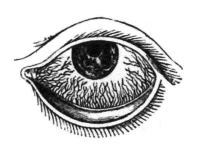

FIG. 52.—Conjunctival congestion. (After Guthrie.)

Symptoms. — 1. **Congestion** of the palpebral and ocular conjunctiva, the pericorneal zone remaining normal or the last part to become red. (Fig. 52.)

2. **Pain** of a scratchy, burning kind, feeling often as if there was a foreign body under the lids.

3. **Vision** slightly diminished owing to the presence of mucus and pus on the cornea.

4. **Discharge** of a muco-purulent nature which mats the lashes into small bundles and sticks the lids together during sleep.

5. **Photophobia** or intolerance of light.

6. Swelling of the lids (slight) and some thickening of the conjunctiva.

Cause. — Foul atmosphere, dust, smoke, wind, heat, cold, the glare of the sun, and errors of refraction. The exanthematous fevers, diseases of the lacrymal sac and duct, nasal catarrh and hay fever. A very contagious form of catarrhal conjunctivitis, which at times becomes epidemic, is caused by a small bacillus described by Weeks; and a conjunctivitis clinically very similar to that produced by the Weeks bacillus is due to the pneumococcus. Also a mild but persistent form of catarrhal conjunctivitis is associated with the presence of the diplo-bacillus of Morax and Axenfeld.

Treatment. — Remove the cause if discovered. Rest eyes and keep them clean. Use a cold compress as follows: —

R

Acidi Borici	3i
Tincturae Opii deodoratae	3vi
Aquae destellatae, q. s. ft.	℥viii

This is to be applied to the outside of the closed lids, on a thin cloth, folded once or twice, for fifteen minutes at a time, four times a day. The solution should be ice cold when used and the wet cloth changed every minute. Apply a weak yellow oxid of mercury ointment or boric acid salve to the edge of the lids at night to prevent adhesion. If discharge is profuse or purulent, paint everted lids, once a day, with a solution of nitrate of silver, five to ten grains to the ounce, or a 2 to 5 per cent solution of protargol. Astringent collyria containing sulfate of zinc, tannin, alum, etc., are very popular. They are, in my estimation, not as useful as the above harmless application and are capable of mischief if, through an error of diagnosis, they are used in iritis, cyclitis or acute keratitis.

An exception should be made of the diplo-bacillus conjunctivitis, in which form sulfate of zinc is particularly valuable.

CHRONIC CATARRHAL CONJUNCTIVITIS.

Symptoms. — After the subsidence of an acute attack the same general symptoms may persist in a milder form, or they may develop slowly without an acute manifestation. In the chronic form the palpebral conjunctiva and the fornix are the parts chiefly involved.

Cause. — The same agents which produce acute catarrhal conjunctivitis, but especially those which are slow and continuous in their action.

Treatment. — The source of any chronic irritation should be removed and the same line of treatment as recommended for an acute attack instituted. Stronger remedies are more applicable to the chronic form, and zinc, alum, nitrate of silver, protargol or sulfate of copper may be used. Caution should be observed in the continuous use of the silver preparations owing to the danger of *argyria*.

PURULENT CONJUNCTIVITIS.

This condition may be divided into two forms: 1. The infantile variety or *Ophthalmia Neonatorum*, which arises between the third and eighth day after birth and generally attacks both eyes. 2. The adult variety, or *Gonorrheal Ophthalmia*, which may attack but one eye.

Symptoms. — The period of incubation varies from 6 to 60 hours. The disease may be divided into three stages: Stage of infiltration, which lasts from 3 to 6 days; stage of pyorrhea, which lasts from 3 to 6 weeks, and stage of chronic blenorrhea, which varies greatly in duration.

1. **Congestion** of the palpebral and ocular conjunctiva.
2. **Pain** is severe and of a smarting, burning variety.

The great thickness and weight of the lids causes also a continuous dull ache in the eye.

3. **Discharge** is profuse and of a thin ichorous, beef juice kind in the first stage which changes in the second to thick yellow pus.

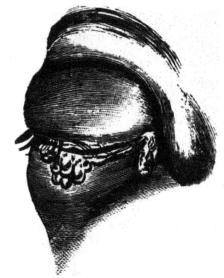

FIG. 53. — Purulent conjunctivitis. (After Dalrymple.)

4. **Swelling** of the lids is so intense as to interfere with the proper inspection of the eye. When the pus begins to flow freely this swelling abates. The conjunctiva becomes so edematous (chemosis) as to overlap the circumference of the cornea.

5. **Vision** may be interfered with by the pus on the cornea, by corneal ulceration, or by the inability to raise the upper lid.

6. **Ulceration of the cornea,** the result of disturbed nutrition and infection, may supervene. This is the most dangerous symptom owing to the possibility of permanent scars, intra-ocular infection, and panophthalmitis.

Cause. — Inoculation with gonorrheal virus, the gono-coccus of Neisser being found in the discharge. There are mild types which clinically simulate purulent conjunctivitis in which the gonococcus cannot be demonstrated. If the gonococcus is absent in the infantile variety, the disease has been caused by a vaginal discharge other than gonorrheal. Such cases are always mild. If the gonococcus is absent in the adult form, the disease must be due to other pus-producing germs. It will sometimes follow mechanical and chemical accidents or badly treated catarrhal conjunctivitis.

Treatment. — In the stage of infiltration cold applications must be kept on the eye continuously. This may be done by keeping a number of small squares of muslin on a block of ice, and transferring one to the eye every minute. The secretion should be washed away with a warm boric acid solution (3 per cent), or some other mild antiseptic, about once every hour. The bowels should be well purged with salines and the patient kept as quiet as possible. If pain is very severe an adult may be given an anodyne. In the stage of pyorrhea the mechanical cleansing of the conjunctiva must be vigorously continued. The upper lid should be turned once a day and its conjunctival surface painted with a 2 per cent solution of nitrate of silver or 20 per cent solution of protargol. If the swelling of the lids is so great as to prevent eversion or to endanger the circulation a canthotomy may be done. In the second stage cold applications should be diminished, if not altogether discontinued, owing to their depressing influence upon the nutrition of the cornea. If the cornea becomes hazy or shows a spot of ulceration hot applications should be applied, for 15 minutes at a time, 4 or 5 times a day; atropin or eserin dropped in the eye and the general treatment for corneal ulcers (page 95) followed as closely as is possible under the circumstances. In the third stage of the disease the treatment advised for chronic catarrhal conjunctivitis (page 71) should be followed.

In adults, where one eye is affected, protect the good eye by covering it with a water crystal held in position by adhesive plaster. To prevent ophthalmia neonatorum in a child born of a diseased mother, resort to the method of Credé, which is to wash its eyes thoroughly just after birth and drop between the lids, several drops of a ten grain to the ounce solution of nitrate of silver.

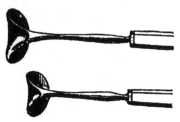

FIG. 54.—Desmarre's elevators used to raise the lids (for inspection of the eye_ball), when they are thick and swollen, as in purulent conjunctivitis.

MEMBRANOUS CONJUNCTIVITIS.

The characteristic feature of this inflammation is a plastic, fibrinous, pseudo-membrane on the tarsal and sometimes on the ocular conjunctiva. With the exception of this membrane the symptoms are very similar to those of purulent conjunctivitis. It is customary to divide this affection into *croupous* and *diphtheritic* conjunctivitis but since the disease appears in every degree of severity, from an almost harmless condition to one of a most destructive character, it is difficult to draw a dividing line clinically. Usually the croupous form is a mild disease, rarely results in any permanent injury and runs a chronic course, while diphtheritic conjunctivitis is acute, severe and destructive. However nothing but the presence of the Klebs-Löffler bacillus will enable us to make a positive differentiation. The disease is rare.

Symptoms. — 1. **Congestion** of the conjunctival vessels is hidden by the plastic membrane in severe cases. In a mild case, the plastic membrane being confined to the lids, the ocular conjunctiva will appear injected.

2. **Pain** is generally of an itching, burning character, but when there is great swelling of the lid there is an added sensation of pressure on the ball.

3. **Discharge** is at first serous and flaky, and may be tinged with a little blood. As soon as the membrane begins to soften the discharge becomes purulent.

4. **Swelling** of the lids is almost imperceptible in the mild forms but in a severe diphtheritic conjunctivitis the upper lid may become so thick and tense as to render its eversion impossible. The exudation into the conjunctiva may be so excessive as to shut off the circulation, producing grangene and subsequent cicatricial contraction and adhesions.

5. **Vision** is affected as in purulent conjunctivitis (page 72).

6. **Ulceration of the cornea** is produced as in purulent conjunctivitis (page 72). In croupous conjunctivitis it rarely happens but in diphtheritic conjunctivitis, if severe, it is almost inevitable.

7. **The membrane** in mild cases is limited to the palpebral conjunctiva and can be wiped off leaving a slightly bleeding surface. In severe cases it covers the entire conjunctiva and can only be removed by force, leaving a raw surface.

8. **Constitutional symptoms** will only be present when the disease is diphtheritic.

Cause. — When the Klebs-Löffler bacillus can be demonstrated the nature of the disease and its cause are definitely determined. The exact cause of those cases in which this bacillus cannot be demonstrated is, as yet, unknown.

Treatment. — For mild cases follow the treatment recommended for catarrial conjunctivitis (page 70) being careful though not to use nitrate of silver until the membrane has disappeared. Before the separation of the membrane cleansing the conjunctival sac three or four times a day with an antiseptic solution (bichlorid 1 to 5,000) is advised. In the severe form follow the treatment as suggested for purulent conjunctivitis (page 73) except that cold applications must not be used as continuously owing to greater danger of depressing the circulation, and nitrate of silver must be applied with caution and then not until the membrane has been thrown off. If the diphtheritic bacillus can be demonstrated constitutional treatment, including antitoxin injections, should be instituted at once.

DISEASES OF THE CONJUNCTIVA (*Continued*).

GRANULAR CONJUNCTIVITIS OR TRACHOMA.

The characteristic feature of this disease is hypertrophy of the conjunctiva and the appearance in that membrane of small granular bodies. Trachoma may assume three forms:—

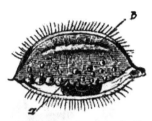

FIG. 55.—Granular upper lid. a, granulations; b, line of scar, in typical position parallel with border of lid. (Nettleship.)

1. **Papillary trachoma** in which the characteristic feature is hypertrophy of the conjunctiva. The normal papillae are greatly increased in size, hence the name. This form is also called chronic conjunctival blenorrhea, as there is always a variable amount of pus in the discharge. Notwithstanding the absence of the trachoma follicles the conjunctiva undergoes cicatricial changes and the sequellae are practically the same as when the granules are present.

2. **Granular trachoma** in which the characteristic feature is the appearance in the conjunctiva of small follicles or granules. These follicles are composed of lymphoid cells and connective tissue cells surrounded by an ill-defined fibrous capsule. They are imbedded in the fibrous layer and have a yellowish or grayish appearance. They develop later into connective tissue which undergoes cicatri-

cial contraction. The follicles are most numerous in the
fornix, but may be found in any part of the palpebral conjunctiva.

3. **Mixed trachoma,** which is the form under which we
generally see the disease, is a combination of the two preceding varieties.

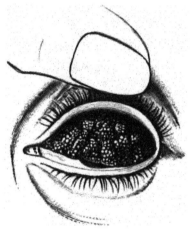

FIG. 56.—Exuberant granulations. No indications of cicatrization are present.
(Jones.)

Symptoms. — The eyes are irritable, giving distress
under exposure or misuse. The lids may be swollen and
may droop a little. There is a slight muco-purulent or
purulent discharge and there is a scratchy feeling under
the lids. Upon inspection of the palpebral conjunctiva the
characteristic appearance above described will be found.
If the disease is of the papillary form the conjunctiva will
have a rough or velvety appearance due to the enlarged
papillae and the color of the swollen conjunctiva is of a
slightly bluish tinge. There will also be some pus in the
conjunctival fornix. If the disease is of the granular form
the peculiar follicles will be present, but as stated above,
the usual picture is a combination of these varieties. With
the progress of the disease all the symptoms increase in
severity. Cicatricial changes will take place in the con-

junctiva and even in the underlying tarsus, rendering the
mucous membrane hard and fibrous in parts and by its
contraction bending the tarsus so as to produce trichiasis
and its attendant evils. The ocular conjunctiva will become injected and *pannus* will develop (page 97). Ulceration of the cornea is a frequent complication and iritis may
occur. Trachoma exhibits a marked tendency toward
remissions and relapses. As a rule the disease covers a
period of years unless persistently and successfully treated.
Some cases seem incurable; they will relapse until vision is
practically destroyed.

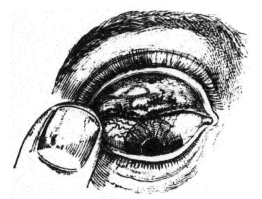

FIG. 57.—Trachoma and pannus. (Berry.)

Cause. — Trachoma is generally conceded to be contagious, and the principle of the contagium is supposed to be
a micro-organism. Numerous trachoma germs have been
described, but none of them has as yet been accepted as the
specific cause of the disease. The fact that one eye may
be affected for years without infecting its fellow is adduced
as an argument against the contagious theory. The tendency of the disease to spread in crowded institutions is
in favor of this theory. Certain races, among which are
the Jews and the Irish, show a predisposition to trachoma,
whereas the negro of our Southern States is almost
immune.

Treatment. — Nitrate of silver, ten grains to the ounce, applied to the conjunctiva once a day or every other day, depending upon the effect, is a valuable remedy. Bichlorid of mercury solution (1 to 4,000) applied directly to the conjunctival surface, is also useful. These two remedies are particularly applicable to the treatment of papillary trachoma. For cases in which the follicular feature predominates, the sulphate of copper stick is the best remedy. This should be applied lightly or thoroughly, daily or with longer intervals, depending upon the effect in each case. In mixed cases it is well to first reduce the papillary swelling with nitrate of silver or bichlorid of mercury and then treat the granular trachoma with bluestone. In the late cicatricial stages ointments of yellow oxid of mercury (grains iv to the ounce) or corrosive sublimate (gr., $\frac{1}{20}$ to the ounce) are recommended. Boroglycerid (30 per cent) and glycerole of tannin (5 to 25 per cent) may be tried.

Where the appearance of the granules indicates its feasibility, squeezing them out with Knapp's roller forceps facilitates the cure. This should be thoroughly done under an anesthetic, and the lids subsequently treated with bichlorid of mercury solution. Old cases, in which there is considerable pannus, as shown in Fig. 56, are often greatly improved by the use of an infusion of jequirity. The cases on which jequirity is used should be carefully selected and as its use is sometimes attended with danger, this treatment should be left to an oculist.

ACUTE TRACHOMA.

During the course of a chronic trachoma the diseased eyes may take on a severe acute inflammation or the disease may seem to originate with an acute attack. Such an inflammation is spoken of as acute trachoma but is in reality a case of chronic trachoma plus an acute conjunctivitis.

Symptoms. — Rapid swelling of the lids and hypertrophy of the conjunctiva. Pain, which may extend to the brow and temples, lacrymation, heat, photophobia and congestion, with a muco-purulent discharge. The palpebral conjunctiva is swollen, red and shiny. The translucent granules, that are covered by the hypertrophied epithelium, usually are not seen until the acute symptoms subside. This occurs in from one to three weeks. It will often be impossible to distinguish this disease from acute catarrhal conjunctivitis until the granules appear.

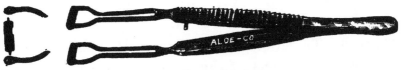

FIG. 58. — Knapp's roller forceps.

Treatment. — Apply iced compresses. Cocain locally is beneficial, but some cases reject it. Distress will sometimes be so great as to warrant the use of bromids or morphin. When the swelling and pain have subsided and the granules appear, treat as a case of chronic trachoma.

FOLLICULAR CONJUNCTIVITIS.

This disease is sometimes described as a form of trachoma, as they are frequently almost identical in appearance. That there is a distinct difference is proven by the fact that follicular conjunctivitis never permanently injures the conjunctiva, whereas trachoma always does.

Symptoms. — The symptoms are those of an acute or chronic catarrhal conjunctivitis to which is added the appearance of the follicles in the fornix of the lower lid, rarely in the upper lid. These granules, about the size of a pin head, are composed of adenoid tissue, identical with that of the true trachoma follicle. They may be few in number or very numerous; if the latter, they are usually arranged in longitudinal rows. The disease is most frequent in children and young people and is very prolonged and obstinate in its course. At times it gives so little annoyance that its presence is discovered by accident.

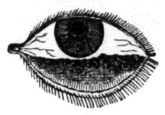

FIG. 59.—Follicular conjunctivitis. (After Eble.)

Cause. — The etiology is obscure. It is supposed to be contagious as so many of the inmates of schools and institutions are attacked at the same time. Bad hygienic surroundings seem to be factors in the production of the disease.

Treatment. — The same treatment as advised for acute or chronic catarrhal conjunctivitis is applicable. An ointment of acetate of lead (gr. i to ℥i) is recommended but acetate of lead must never be used if there is any implication of the cornea. If the follicles are prominent, expression with the roller forceps will hasten the cure. Fresh air, good food, proper exercise, attention to refractive errors and the proper use of the eyes must not be overlooked.

DISEASES OF THE CONJUNCTIVA (*Continued*).

PTERYGIUM.

This is a triangular mass of hypertrophied conjunctiva, the apex of which encroaches upon the cornea, with the base generally toward the inner, sometimes toward the outer canthus. In rare instances an eye may have two pterygia, one on each side. The head or apex is firmly united to the cornea, sometimes going deep enough to destroy the membrane of Bowman. A pterygium rarely

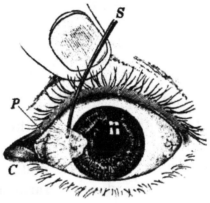

FIG. 60.—Pterygium. C, caruncle; P, punctum; S, probe passed under the upper margin. (Fuchs.)

grows beyond the center of the cornea and usually it requires years for the apex to reach that point. While progressing a pterygium is red, fleshy and vascular (p. crassum), later, development ceases and it becomes thin, white, membranous and more or less bloodless (p. tenue). It affects vision by growing in front of the pupil or by traction producing astigmatism.

Cause.—It is found usually in those whose eyes are subjected to the irritation of wind and weather. Fuchs claims it is developed from a pinguecula, others maintain that its starting-point is an erosion of the corneal limbus. Laymen will usually call this growth cataract.

Treatment is operative. *False pterygium* partakes of the character of a symblepharon. It is an inflammatory adhesion of the ocular conjunctiva to a denuded or ulcerated point of the corneal limbus which is the result of acute blenorrhea, diphtheria, burns or injury. It can be differentiated from true pterygium by its history, the fact that it may appear at any point on the circumference of the cornea, and that it has no tendency to progress.

PINGUECULA.

This is a small yellow elevation in the conjunctiva, generally found between the limbus of the cornea and the plica semilunaris, but sometimes on the temporal side. It is composed of connective tissue and elastic fibres. It is of frequent occurrence, does no harm and need not be removed.

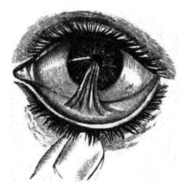

FIG. 61.—Symblepharon. (After Mackenzie.)

SYMBLEPHARON.

This is a cicatricial adhesion between the conjunctiva of the lid and the conjunctiva of the ball and is the result of the apposition of two raw surfaces, which may have been produced by operations, ulcers, burns, etc. The treatment is operative and difficult. After dissecting the lid from the ball the raw surfaces must be thoroughly covered by mucous membrane or they will promptly reunite.

BURNS.

Burns of the conjunctiva are serious because they lead to the adhesion between the lids and globe just described.

Powder burns may only involve the outside of the lids and may, if the eye is not closed quickly enough, seriously damage the cornea and entail loss of sight. The burns of percussion caps and torpedoes are especially destructive, owing to the added evil of the chemical action of the fulminate of silver and mercury of which they are made. All the foreign particles should be carefully picked out of the skin and cornea, an anodyne given to control the pain, and the eye put up in an aseptic oil dressing. If the cornea is much injured atropin should be used, as there is danger of secondary iritis.

Lime burns must be washed copiously with tepid water and all particles picked out with forceps if an anesthetic has to be given to accomplish it. A weak solution of vinegar may be used. An anodyne can be given and cocain used locally. Adhesions should be broken every day and sweet oil dropped between the lids. If the burn is deep symblepharon will follow.

Acid burns should be thoroughly cleansed with weak bicarbonate of soda solution, and the raw surfaces, pain and inflammation combatted as in the case of lime burns. Atropin should always be used where there is danger of iritis.

SUB-CONJUNCTIVAL ECCHYMOSIS.

A hemorrhage under the conjunctiva may be due to a strain, traumatism or disease of the blood vessels. It is seen often in children with whooping cough, and need cause no uneasiness. Coming on in an adult, without strain or accident, it indicates weakness of the vessel walls and portends hemorrhages in other organs, which might be of serious consequence. There is no pain attending the condition and treatment is unnecessary. Hot applications may hasten absorption of the clot.

MORBID GROWTHS IN THE CONJUNCTIVA.

Under this head I will only mention the abnormal growths which may develop, as the diagnosis and treatment of these conditions lie along surgical lines. Syphilitic and tubercular lesions may be found in the conjunctiva, detection of the latter often requiring fine diagnostic discrimination. Epitheliomata and sarcomata may develop, and usually elect the limbus as their starting-point. Thorough removal is imperative. Some cases demand sacrifice of the eyeball and orbital contents but even this does not always save the patient. Lipomata are found under the conjunctiva, between the superior and external rectus muscles and must be differentiated from a dislocated lacrymal gland. Papillomata may grow from any part of the conjunctiva, while Dermoid tumors are, as a rule, found as congenital formations, near the outer canthus. Cysts, Nevi and Angiomata are also found in the conjunctiva.

DISEASES OF THE CORNEA.

PHLYCTENULAR KERATITIS.

Phlyctenular keratitis and phlyctenular conjunctivitis are the same disease, the only difference being in the location of the vesicle. The small blister, which is the characteristic feature of the disease, may be located on the scleral conjunctiva or on the cornea, but is most frequently found between the two, at the limbus. When on the cornea, all the symptoms are more severe than when the disease is conjunctival, and it is only when corneal that it can leave any changes which impair vision. The number of vesicles is not limited, and it is possible to have them on the cornea and conjunctiva at the same time.

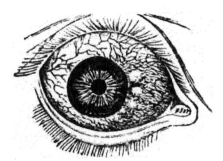

FIG. 62.—Phlyctenular conjunctivitis. (After Dalrymple.)

Symptoms.— The vesicle, a small, red nodule, is at first a circumscribed accumulation of leucocytes, under the epithelial layer, but soon develops into an ulcer. The conjunctiva is injected, and there is a tendency of the enlarged vessels toward the phlyctene. Photophobia and pain are severe, which produces strong blepharospasm. Lacrymation is pronounced. Generally there is a discharge from the nose, and eczematous scabs form around the lips and nostrils. There may be enlargement of the lymphatic glands and other evidences of a strumous diathesis. Usually the disease recovers in a few weeks, leaving no permanent injury, but relapses are the rule. Faint opacities of the cornea may be left, which, if over the pupil, will impair vision. In rare instances deep ulceration of the cornea may develop, followed by secondary iritis, perforation or staphyloma.

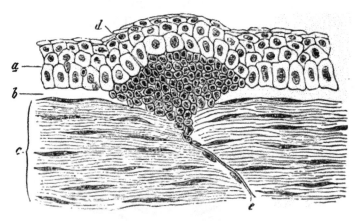

Fig. 63.—Phlyctenular keratitis. a, epithelial layer; b, membrane of Bowman; c, substantia propria; d, accumulation of leucocytes; e, corneal nerve.   (Iwanoff.)

Cause. — It is a disease of childhood, and is supposed to be due to some irregularity of nutrition, the result of the strumous diathesis. Bad hygienic surroundings and insufficient nourishment seem to contribute to the disease, and yet it is frequently seen in otherwise healthy children.

Treatment. — The cause being constitutional, give fresh air, wholesome food, tonics of syrup of the iodid of iron, malt or cod liver oil, and keep bowels regular. Small doses of calomel are efficacious. Promote health in every way. Use locally hot fomentations and a weak ointment of yellow oxid of mercury rubbed in gently once a day. If the disease is limited to the conjunctiva, the cold application advised for conjunctival inflammation (page 70) may be useful. If pronounced corneal ulceration develops, follow the treatment for such a condition (page 95). Constitutional treatment should be continued after the disappearance of the local disease.

INTERSTITIAL KERATITIS.

This is a disease of childhood but may be found in early adult life. The substantia propria is the part primarily involved. The deeper layers soon participate in the inflammation and in severe cases the uveal tract rarely escapes. The course of the disease is generally chronic, sometimes extending over two or three years. The prognosis is favorable, although only a few cases escape without some impairment of vision. In a limited number sight is permanently lost.

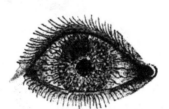

FIG. 64.—Interstitial keratitis. (Nettleship.)

Symptoms.—At first the eye will indicate a state of irritability. There will be some photophobia, lacrymation and circumcorneal hyperemia. Vision will become blurred and inspection will reveal an infiltration of the deeper layers of the cornea, which gives it an opaque or hazy appearance. This haziness may begin in the center or it may start from the scleral margin. Small blood vessels will be seen springing from the corneal periphery and extending towards its center. These blood vessels are deep in the substantia propria and if numerous will give the inflamed area a salmon pink color. The opacity of the cornea may become complete in a short time and vision be reduced to light perception. Iritis may occur with a tendency toward the inflammation extending to the ciliary body and choroid. When resolution sets in the opacity begins to disappear at the margin, the center of the cornea being the last part to become transparent. When the iris can be seen posterior synechiae may be found and when the fundus can be examined we may find evidences of choroidal inflammation. Associated with the eye symptoms we generally find evidences of inherited syphilis; glandular enlargement, sunken nose, ozena, Hutchinson's teeth, scars at the angles of the mouth, the vaulted palate and the characteristic physiognomy.

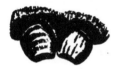 

FIG. 65.—Hutchinson's teeth.

Cause.—Nettleship claims to have found evidences of inherited syphilis in 68 per cent of his cases, and suspects it in the remaining 32 per cent. It is said also to be caused by tuberculosis, rheumatism and acquired syphilis.

Treatment.—Use smoked glasses to protect the eyes from the light. Apply hot applications for thirty minutes at a time three or four times a day. Drop into eyes, twice a day, a one per cent solution of sulfate of atropin. Assume the existence of syphilis and give anti-syphilitic remedies with tonics, good food and good air. After the acute symptoms have subsided use a weak ointment of the yellow oxid of mercury (grs. 2 to ℥i) putting into the conjunctival sac, once a day, a quantity about half the size of a pea. The ointment can be thoroughly disseminated, and at the same time a massage of the cornea effected, by placing a finger on the closed lid and giving it a gentle lateral or rotary movement. Dusting the cornea with calomel has been recommended, but it must be remembered that calomel should never be put into an eye when the patient is taking iodid of potassium, as the iodid is found in the tears and with the colomel makes an intensely irritating compound. If the massage with the yellow oxid of mercury ointment or the dusting with colomel causes undue reaction, it indicates that the remedy has been employed too soon and its use should be postponed until the eyes are less sensitive.

Non suppurative Keratitis
1. Stage of Infiltration
2. " of Suppuration

Suppuration
Infiltration
Suppuration { Progressive
{ Regressive
Cicatrization

Examine Corneal reflex. If the surface
see it is ___ . If loss of substance
dealing with a foul ulcer. If the
lustrous the affection is an old one.
no of substance it is a clean ulcer. If
no of substance you have a cicatrix.

DISEASES OF THE CORNEA (*Continued*).

ULCERATION OF THE CORNEA.

Symptoms. — Congestion, pain, lacrymation, impairment of vision and swelling of the lids are associated with ulceration of the cornea, but the latter, being due to such a diversity of causes, will show a great variety of symptomatic pictures. For example, an eye with ulceration of the

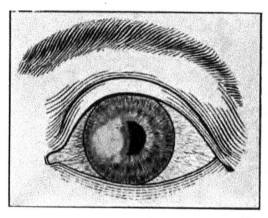

FIG. 66. — A large superficial ulcer of the cornea. The ulcer is surrounded by a zone of infiltration.

cornea resulting from diphtheritic conjunctivitis will necessarily present a very different appearance from one in which the ulcer is due to an infected foreign body. Corneal ulcers have also been accurately classified according to shape, method of development and cause, but for the purposes of the student a general description is deemed sufficient.

The part of the cornea involved becomes infiltrated and appears hazy, white or yellow. This is quickly followed by a loss of corneal substance. The destruction of tissue may spread superficially or may involve the deeper layers and result in speedy perforation. The ulcer will be surrounded by a hazy zone of infiltrated tissue, the region of densest infiltration corresponding to the direction in which the ulcer is most liable to progress. If the disintegrating process only involves the first two layers, repair with transparent tissue will result, but any loss of the deeper layers will be replaced by an opaque scar. An ulcer will meet with greater resistance from the membrane of Descemet

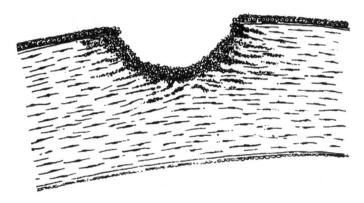

FIG. 67.—Ulcer of the cornea. The epithelium, Bowman's membrane and part of the substantia propria are gone. The floor of the ulcer is infiltrated with pus cells.

than from any other layer of the cornea, and is often checked at this point. If Descemet's membrane gives way, perforation follows. When this takes place the aqueous escapes and the iris and lens come forward to the cornea. If the iris adheres permanently to the corneal cicatrix, we have a condition called *anterior synechia*. Contact of the anterior lens capsule with the cornea is liable to produce an opacity of the capsule at the point of contact if the patient be very young. When the aqueous escapes the tension is relieved and the lymph circulation in the cornea becomes freer, which accounts for the improvement so often noted after perforation. Iritis occurs frequently and is sure to occur if the deeper layers of the cornea are involved. Adhesion of the iris to the lens capsule or *posterior synechia* must be guarded against. The ciliary body may become involved. In some cases there is an exudation of non-pathogenic pus from the iris which forms at the bottom of the anterior chamber. Pus in the anterior chamber is called *hypopyon*. The presence of hypopyon adds gravity to the disease, and in such cases the prognosis should be extremely guarded. The entire cornea may melt away and the eyeball still be preserved by the formation of a white, fibrous cicatrix where the cornea was. This new tissue may not be as resisting as the cornea, and is liable to be protruded by the intra-ocular pressure, causing *staphyloma* (page 98). After perforation intra-ocular infection may occur and the eye be destroyed by *panophthalmitis* (page 113).

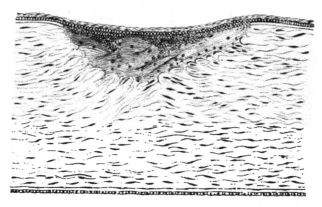

FIG. 68. — The cornea after ulceration, showing the scar tissue.

Cause. — The *exciting* cause is a pathogenic microbe, generally the white or yellow staphylococci, the pneumococcus or the streptococcus. The source of the germ may be purulent conjunctivitis, dacryocystitis, erysipelas, diphtheria, ozena, septic fingers, handkerchiefs and instruments, or an unknown source.

The *predisposing* cause is some condition which renders the cornea more susceptible to infection. This may be a debilitating disease, an injury from a foreign body, an operation, lagophthalmia (paralysis of the seventh nerve), or paralysis of the fifth nerve. The ulceration due to paralysis of the fifth is called *neuroparalytic keratitis*. With paralysis of the fifth there is loss of sensation, foreign bodies are no longer removed from the cornea, by the reflex action of the lids, and abrasion results. Abrasion is further facilitated by the dryness of the cornea which exists in the absence of winking.

Treatment. — When the ulcer is due to purulent conjunctivitis, dacryocystitis erysipelas, diphtheria, etc., the primary disease must be treated vigorously. If the secretion is scant the lids should be immobilized, between treatments, by a light bandage, if abundant the bandage should not be used. The focus of germs should be destroyed by touching the ulcer with a galvanic cautery, tincture of iodin or carbolic acid, or by scraping it clean with a small curette. This should be done under holocain (one per cent), anesthesia. Holocain is preferable to cocain as it does not dry the corneal epithelium, and also possesses some antiseptic properties. The conjunctival sac should be cleansed out about three times a day with bichlorid of mercury solution 1 to 5000. The cleansing may be repeated more frequently if a saturated solution of boracic acid or biborate of soda is used. The direct application of a strong protargol solution (20 per cent) has been extolled. Hot fomentations should be applied for thirty minutes at a time every three hours. About three times a day instil a drop of a one per cent solution of atropin to relieve iritic congestion and prevent posterior synechia. Some advise the use of eserin to relieve intra-ocular tension and thus improve the lymph circulation in the cornea. but this is manifestly dangerous if the iris is involved. The local application of a 10 per cent ointment of cassareep is said to relieve pain and otherwise favorably influence the disease. Paracentesis will relieve the tension and is sometimes indicated, especially if perforation is imminent.

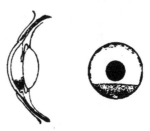

FIG. 69. — Hypopyon, seen from the front, and in section, to show that the pus is behind the cornea. (Nettleship.)

The patient should be kept quiet and the constitution sustained by iron, quinin, and strychnin tonics. If the ulceration is neuroparalytic or is due to paralysis of the seventh nerve, the cornea must be protected by the lid and a bandage or adhesive plaster will be necessary to accomplish it.

Forms. 1. Superficial. 2. Deep ? Keratitis ?
3. Pannus.

ial

ising from network of marginal
the limbus & can be followed into
Conjunctiva.

al position clear, well
& color.

branch in abonement

al surface uneven because
raise epithelial
mation & injection of
oedema of conjunctivas &
Inflamed,
, may organize & close

Deep.

1. Vessels spring from
close to marginal
? appear to end at
Limbus as they do
behind it.

2. Indistinct, diffe
colon rety & greyish
because come old by e
layers.

3. Fine twigs & run

4. Corneal surface
& lusterless

5. Inflamatrio &
of ovessels. 6
conjunctiva & lid
Hyplopion

DISEASES OF THE CORNEA (*Cont'd*) AND SCLERA.

VASCULAR KERATITIS OR PANNUS.

The u))er 1alf of the cornea is the)art most frequentl)
affected, but its w1ole surface may be involved. It becomes grayish in color from cellular infiltration and covered b) a mes1 of fine blood vessels, w1ic1 grow from the
conjunctiva. The infiltration and vascularity are found between the e)it1elial and Bowman's layers, but may go

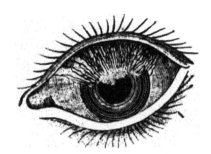

FIG. 70. — 1annus. (Fick.)

dee)er. If the new growt1 invades the substantia)ro)ria
permanent scarring is the result. Vision is im)aired and
may be reduced to lig1t)erception. As)annus is secondary to some ot1er ocular disease the general symptoms
will be t1ose of the)rimar) affection.

Cause. — Long-continued irritation of the cornea from
trac1oma, man) considering it the onl) cause of true pannus,)ersistent)1l)ctenular keratitis, ingrowing las1es,
ex)osure from im)erfect closure of the lids, etc.

Treatment. — Attend to the primary disease. The use
of an infusion of jequirit))roduces a severe and dangerous

 purulent inflammation, which often results in great improvement and sometimes cure of the pannus, but this treatment should be left to an oculist.

OPACITIES OF THE CORNEA.

Nebula, macula and leucoma are names given to opacities of the cornea. These opacities represent scar tissue, which has replaced the loss of substance occasioned by an ulcer. If the first two layers of the cornea are destroyed they may heal without leaving any sign, but any loss of the deeper layers is repaired with scar tissue. The amount of damage to sight produced by an opacity depends upon its location relative to the pupil. Recent scars are improved by time and direct massage with a stimulating ointment, but old ones will remain unchanged. If the opacity is central and there is any peripheral clear cornea, an artificial pupil may improve vision. Before advising an iridectomy it is wise to dilate the pupil to the maximum extent and observe if this measure improves vision; if not, a false pupil will be of little service.

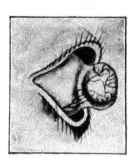

FIG. 71.—Total staphyloma. (Fick.)

STAPHYLOMA.

Severe ulceration of the cornea so decreases its power of resistance that the normal intra-ocular pressure may cause it to bulge forward, destroying the natural curve. The distension may involve the whole cornea or only part of it. When staphyloma is the result of a perforating ulcer, the iris may be caught in its tissue and severe pain and intra-ocular inflammation result. The staphylomatous cornea is never transparent. It may be stationary or progressive. It may be small or so large that the lids will not close over it. In some cases nothing need be done. The treatment is operative.

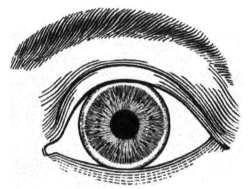

FIG. 72. — An arcus senilis.

ARCUS SENILIS.

A narrow white ring is often seen near the circumference of the cornea. It is usually found in old people but may occur in the young. It is caused by hyaline degeneration and requires no treatment. It has no influence on the healing of wounds, as for example the incision in cataract operation.

CONICAL CORNEA.

Sometimes the center of the cornea becomes weakened by an atrophic process and the intra-ocular pressure pushes it forward; the convex sphere changing to a cone. The cornea remains clear except for the occasional appearance of a nebula at its apex. The process is slow and gradual but finally reaches a point where it stops. Vision is greatly impaired.   Inspection of the eye reveals no abnormality, except in pronounced cases, when a side view will

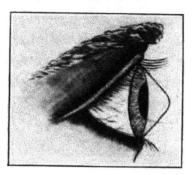

FIG. 73—A conical cornea.

show its conical form.   Diagnosis in the early stages is difficult and treatment not very effective.   The latter should be left to an oculist.

FOREIGN BODIES IN THE CORNEA.

It is very common for cinders, sand, pieces of emory, iron, steel, etc., to become lodged in the cornea.   Pain and lacrymation will be intense, with more or less circumcorneal injection.   If simple inspection does not reveal the offender use oblique illumination.   This is done by seating the patient about two feet from a light and with a 16 or 20 Dioptre convex lens, focus the rays *obliquely* on the part to be examined.   In this way the cornea, iris and anterior part of the lens may be thoroughly inspected.   To remove a foreign body, the cornea should first be anesthetized by several drops of a 4 per cent solution of cocain or a 1 per cent solution of holocain; then, with a needle or spud pick it out with as little destruction to corneal tissue as possible. When the epithelium is denuded there is always danger of infection; therefore, an antiseptic collyrium (solution hydrarg. bichlorid 1 to 5,000) should be used for three or four days, or until the epithelial layer is restored. Another way to prevent infection of the cornea when the epithelium has been denuded, is to touch the lesion lightly with compound tincture of benzoin. A thin, adherent pellicle is immediately formed, which covers the wound for from six to twelve hours.

DISEASES OF THE SCLERA.

EPISCLERITIS.

Under the ocular conjunctiva is a delicate membrane, the capsule of Tenon and between the capsule of Tenon and the sclera proper is the loose connective tissue called the episclera. These parts are so intimately related that inflammation of the subconjunctival tissues generally involves the overlying conjunctiva and may go deeper into the sclera proper. Scleral and episcleral inflammation is limited to the region anterior to the equator.

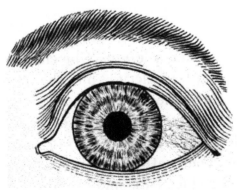

FIG. 74—A schematic representation of the nodule and patch of injection in a case of episcleritis.

Symptoms. — In episcleritis there appears a patch of dusky red injection under the conjunctiva, generally between the insertion of a rectus muscle and the cornea. There may be a distinct nodule which will tend to confound the disease with phlyctenular conjunctivitis. The age of the patient and the fact that the episcleral nodule does not ulcerate will aid in the differentiation. The discharge from the eye is watery and pain and photophobia are generally slight. The inflamed spot may disappear spontaneously, may persist for weeks, has a tendency to recur, and will often leave a gray, discolored patch.

Cause. — Rheumatism, gout, scrofula, syphilis and menstrual derangement. It may arise from exposure to the weather and is also said to appear over the insertion of a rectus muscle suffering from insufficiency. Frequently the cause is obscure.

Treatment. — Some cases are so mild as to need no treatment. The constitutional cause, if discoverable, should be attended to. Correct muscular anomalies and refractive errors. Apply hot fomentation. Use atropin if there is any tendency toward iritis. When chronic, stimulation with yellow oxid of mercury ointment is useful.

SCLERITIS.

Inflammation of the sclera may be circumscribed or diffuse. It resembles episcleritis but the symptoms are all more severe and, as a deeper structure is inflamed, there is much greater danger of involvement of the uvea. The discharge is watery and pain and photophobia may be pronounced. The inflammation may extend to the underlying uveal tract and produce iritis and cyclitis; or extend to the cornea, producing a haziness of its deep layers (sclero keratitis.) The condition is usually chronic, sometimes extending over a period of years. The scleral wall may become thinned and staphyloma follow.

Cause. — The cause is generally rheumatism, gout, syphilis, scrofula or menstrual disorders.

Treatment. — For the syphilitic form use mercury and iodid of potassium. In scrofulous cases, tonics, good air and good food. When due to rheumatism, salicylate of sodium, Rochelle salts, etc. If gouty in origin, iodid of potassium or colchicum. Combine above treatment with hot baths, warm fomentations over eyes, leeching of the temples, and locally, cocain and atropin. Never put irritants, such as zinc or copper in these eyes.

DISEASES OF THE IRIS.

Mydriasis or dilatation of the pupil may be due to many causes, among which are: —

1. The use of drugs called mydriatics, such as atropin, homatropin, scopolamin and cocain. Most mydriatics also produce paralysis of accommodation.
2. Increase of intra-ocular pressure as in glaucoma.
3. Loss of vision as in atrophy of the optic nerve.
4. Paralysis of the third nerve.
5. Dimness of light.
6. Ingestion of certain drugs, belladonna, ergot, etc.
7. Apoplexia in the later stages.

Myosis or contraction of the pupil may be due to: —

1. The use of drugs called myotics, such as eserin and pilocarpin. The myotics also stimulate accommodation.
2. Evacuation of the aqueous humor.
3. Hyperemia of the iris as in iritis.
4. Paralysis of the cervical sympathetic nerve.
5. Bright light, accommodation and convergence.
6. Ingestion of certain drugs, as opium and alcohol.
7. Apoplexia in the early stages.

The Argyll-Robertson pupil is one which responds to convergence but not to light, and is significant of locomotor ataxia. The variations of mydriasis and myosis dependent upon irritation and disease of the brain and spinal cord are too complex to dwell upon here.

Anterior synechia is an adhesion of the iris to the cornea, due to perforation of the cornea and lodgment of the iris in the wound.

Posterior synechia is an adhesion of the iris to the anterior capsule of the lens. In complete posterior synechia

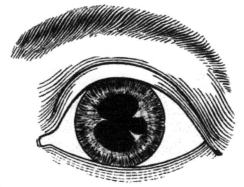

FIG. 75.— Posterior synechia. Adhesion of the iris to the anterior capsule of the lens at three points.

we have what is called *exclusion* of the pupil. Where the pupillary area is filled by a membrane, we have *occlusion* of the pupil. (Fig. 76)

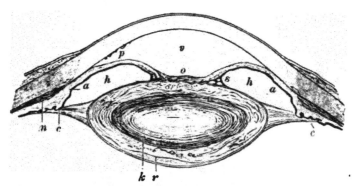

FIG. 76.—Exclusion and occlusion of the pupil, with bulging of the iris forward from accumulation of fluid in the posterior chamber. The posterior chamber (h) is thus made deeper, the anterior chamber (v) shallower, especially where the root of the iris (a) is pressed against the cornea. The pupil is closed by an exudate membrane o. (Fuchs.)

IRITIS.

The disease may be divided by its course into acute or chronic; pathologically it may be plastic, suppurative or serous; etiologically it may be divided into as many forms as there are causes, the leading varieties being syphilitic, rieumatic, gouty, idiopatiic, traumatic and secondary. The typical form of iritis, is)lastic; serous iritis, according to Collins, Priestley Smiti and otiers, being more a))ro)riately a cyclitis.

PLASTIC IRITIS.

Symptoms. — Injection of the dee) blood vessels around the cornea, later extending over the entire wiite of the eye. Disciarge of a watery ciaracter. Intolerance of ligit and pain of a neuralgic nature, beginning in the eyeball and extending over the brow, tem)les and cheek. The)u)il becomes small and will not react to ligit. Its normal color changes to a darker tone, a blue or gray iris becoming green. The aqueous becomes turbid from lym)ioid cells, pus and red blood corpuscles, and vision is corres)ondingly im)aired. Adiesion will take)lace between the iris and anterior lens capsule, constituting posterior synechia. If tiese adhesions are broken,)igment de)osits will be left on the capsule of the lens. Wien the

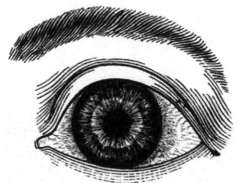

FIG. 77.—Circumcorneal injection, the deep blood vessels around the limbus being the ones involved.

attack is sy)iilitic in origin, gummata may develo) on the iris. If tiere is muci pus in the aqueous humor it may settle in the anterior ciamber,)roducing hypopium.

Sometimes the exudation in the anterior ciamber leaves

a membrane across the pupil which may be mistaken for cataract. Such a condition is spoken of as occlusion of the pupil. (Fig. 76.) Iritis may attack one eye or both. Its duration depends largely upon the treatment, but will generally last from two to six weeks. In some cases the eye will be myopic for weeks after an attack of iritis.

Cause. — In fifty per cent of all cases it is due to syphilis, secondary, tertiary, acquired or inherited. The next most potent factors are rheumatism and gout. It may arise as secondary to other eye diseases or be due to direct lesion, accidental or operative. Gonorrhœa and diabetes are also said to be etiological factors.

Treatment. — Prohibit work and protect eyes with shaded glasses. Look to the general health of patient, paying special attention to the condition of the alimentary canal. To prevent posterior synechia, dilate pupil with atropin and keep it dilated through the whole attack. Leeching at the temple is sometimes efficacious. For the pain, give antipyrin or morphin and apply heat, dry or in the form of watery fomentation. In syphilitic cases give mercury and iodid of potassium. When rheumatic or gouty in origin, use the salicylates, colchicum, lithia, etc., combined with hot baths or pilocarpin sweats.

SUPPURATIVE IRITIS.

This form is generally due to wounds or operations and does not differ materially from the plastic form, except that the presence of pus infection makes the symptoms more severe and the prognosis very grave. It may also be due to infectious diseases, pyæmia and meningitis.

SEROUS IRITIS.

This disease and serous cyclitis are the same; not only are the iris, ciliary body and the choroid involved, but also

Descemet's membrane of the cornea. It has been described under the names descemitis, keratitis postica, keratitis punctata, serous uveitis and serous irido-cyclitis.

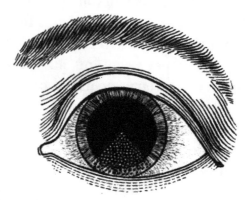

FIG. 78.—Serous iritis, showing ciliary injection and keratitis punctata. Pupil dilated by a mydriatic.

Symptoms. — Slight pericorneal injection, pain insignificant, vision sometimes only a little below normal, but may be much lowered, increase of aqueous evidenced by unusual depth of the anterior chamber and plus tension. The pupil will not be contracted as in plastic iritis and the iris will only be slightly discolored. Posterior synechia may occur, but is not as common as in other forms of iritis. There will also be found a characteristic cellular deposit in the form of fine dots on the lower half of the posterior surface of the cornea, which constitutes *keratitis punctata.* The course of the disease is more or less chronic and the subjective symptoms mild as compared with the other forms of iritis.

Cause. — The causes are the same as

Treatment. — The same as in plastic iritis except that atropin must be carefully used owing to the danger of increasing the tension. If the sion becomes dangerous it may be reduced by the locally, or pilocarpin injectio

DISEASES OF THE CILIARY BODY AND CHOROID.

DISEASES OF THE CILIARY BODY.

Inflammation of the ciliary body is not an isolated condition, but is probably always associated with disease of the iris or choroid. Cyclitis may be acute or chronic; plastic, suppurative or serous.

PLASTIC AND SUPPURATIVE CYCLITIS.

The symptoms of these two conditions are the same as in iritis, with the addition of opacity of the vitreous, severe pain upon pressure over the region of the ciliary body and characteristic tension, which is plus in the acute stage but later becomes decidedly minus, due to atrophy of the ciliary body and shrinkage of the vitreous. The lens sometimes becomes opaque and detachment of the retina may occur. Plastic cyclitis is dangerous, suppurative cyclitis is almost always fatal to vision. Treatment is the same as in iritis.

SEROUS CYCLITIS.

This is the same as serous iritis (page 107).

SYMPATHETIC OPHTHALMIA.

Sympathetic ophthalmia is a diseased condition arising in one eye, caused by some organic lesion of its fellow. The eye which is first affected is called the *exciting* eye, while the other is called the *sympathizing* eye.

The disease takes two forms — sympathetic irritation and sympathetic inflammation.

Symptoms. — (1) Sympathetic irritation is a functional derangement characterized by intolerance of light, lacrymation and fatigue of the eye when used. Visual acuity may be impaired and sometimes temporary obscuration of sight occurs. There may be considerable pain, of a neuralgic character, in and around the eye, and also some pericorneal injection. The symptoms may subside, but a relapse will occur. Unless the exciting eye is enucleated, the disease is prone to develop into sympathetic inflammation.

(2) Sympathetic inflammation is sometimes very slow and insidious in its development. When established there is intense circumcorneal injection, an inflamed iris, contracted pupil, punctate deposits upon Descemet's membrane, lowered vision, opacities in the vitreous, intense neuralgic pain in the region supplied by the fifth nerve; also pain upon pressure over the ciliary region. As the disease progresses optic neuritis, choroiditis, synchisis of the vitreous and detachment of the retina develop.

Cause. — The cause is an inflammation of the uveal tract of the exciting eye. This uveitis may be idiopathic, but the inflammation most prone to excite sympathetic trouble is that due to a wound of the ciliary region or the presence of a foreign body in the exciting eye. Other sources of the exciting uveitis are perforating corneal ulcers and intraocular tumors. After an enucleation the optic nerve or ciliary nerves being caught in the cicatrix have been known to give rise to sympathetic irritation. Sympathetic ophthalmia may arise at any time from two weeks to many years after the lesion of the exciting eye. In spite of many theories our knowledge of how this inflammation is conveyed from one eye to the other is yet speculative.

Treatment. — As sympathetic irritation is always cured by enucleating the exciting eye, this should be done at once, but if sympathetic inflammation is established this procedure will rarely stop it and should not be resorted to if the exciting eye has useful vision, as it will often retain the best vision of the two. If, in sympathetic inflammation, the exciting eye is blind, enucleate it. Its removal may do some good and can do no harm. The patient should be kept in a dark room, hot fomentations used from four to eight hours a day, anodynes given for pain and mercury and tonics given internally. Salicylate of soda to the limit of toleration has been advised. As the treatment of sympathetic inflammation is so unsatisfactory, its prophylaxis becomes doubly important and I would advise the enucleation of all blind eyes affected with chronic irido-cyclitis; all eyes with irido-cyclitis due to the presence of a foreign body, which cannot be removed, even if some vision remains; also all shrunken globes and stumps which are tender on pressure.

DISEASES OF THE CHOROID.

The function of the choroid is to nourish the retina and vitreous, and to prevent reflection, by the power to absorb light possessed by its pigment. In Albinos there is almost a total absence of pigment in the uveal tract, and great distress from photophobia is the result. Albinos are, as a rule, afflicted with amblyopia, refractive errors or nystagmus. Dark glasses are often a necessity to these patients.

CHOROIDITIS.

Symptoms. — If the morbid process is limited to the choroid, external signs of inflammation are absent. Visual

disturbance will be the only subjective symptom, and the
objective symptoms will be revealed by the opthalmoscope.
The visual disturbance will consist of floating bodies in the
field, or of one or more areas, in which vision is reduced or
lost, called scotomata. There may also be distortion of the
outline of objects called metamorphosia. The amount of
disturbance of vision may depend largely upon the proximity of the inflamed area to the macula.

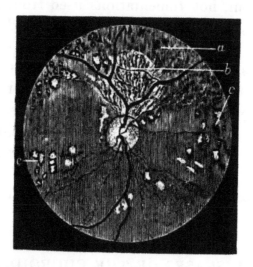

FIG. 79 — Atrophy after syphilitic choroditis, showing various degrees of wasting.
(Hutchinson.) a, atrophy of pigment epithelium: b, atrophy of epithelium and
chorio-capillaris; the large vessels exposed: c, spots of complete atrophy, many
with pigment accumulation.

The opthalmoscope will show, in recent cases, ill-defined
yellowish patches under the retinal vessels. These spots of
exudation may absorb and leave no sign, but generally the
choroid at these points atrophies and the sclera shows
glistening white through it. Around the borders of these
atrophic areas, pigment is soon deposited. The retina over
the inflamed area is usually involved and also partakes of the
subsequent atrophy, which explains the scotomata or blind
spots in the field of vision. The inflammatory process may
extend to the vitreous and cause a cloudiness of that body,

at times so dense as to prevent an opthalmoscopic view of the underlying tissues.

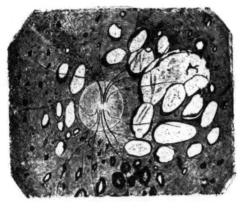

FIG. 80.—Atrophic patches in the choroid (choroiditis disseminata). (After Foerster.)

Cause. — Syphilis, malnutrition, scrofula, anemia and high myopia, and in some cases no cause can be assigned with any degree of accuracy. The choroid being a part of the uveal tract is subject to inflammation arising in the iris and ciliary body.

Treatment. — Absolute rest of eyes and the use of mydriatics, smoked glasses, mercury, iodid of potassium and tonics.

PANOPHTHALMITIS.

This is an acute purulent inflammation of the contents of the globe in which vision is always lost.

Symptoms. — Intense pain, swelling of the lids and chemosis of the conjunctiva, with early loss of vision. There may be a rise in temperature and vomiting. If the process begins in an ulcer or wound of the cornea this tissue will soon become opaque and suppurative. If the lesion starts from within, the iris will change color as in iritis, and the aqueous become muddy, but in spite of this the yellow reflex caused by pus behind the lens may generally be seen.

8

Cause. —Intra-ocular pus infection from wounds, operations, perforating ulcers of the cornea, pyemia by metastasis or meningitis.

Treatment. —Control the pain by leeches, hot bichlorid fomentations and anodynes, and enucleate as soon as convinced that the eye is lost. Evisceration is preferred by some as offering less danger of setting up a purulent meningitis than enucleation.

LESSON XX.

DISEASES OF THE CRYSTALLINE LENS.

DISLOCATION OF THE LENS.

This condition may exist congenitally or may be due to accident or disease. The lens may be partially held by the suspensory ligament or may be totally detached. The dislocation may be to the side, back into the vitreous or forward, through the pupil, into the anterior chamber. If due to disease it is associated with choroiditis, cyclitis and a fluid state of the vitreous. The lens may be perfectly transparent or cataractous. If cataractous the malposition may be easily detected (Fig. 81). If transparent and not

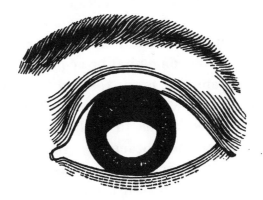

FIG. 81.— Downward dislocation of a cataractous lens.

in the anterior chamber the ophthalmoscope will reveal the condition. A transparent lens in the anterior chamber can be diagnosed by close inspection with the unaided eye. Congenital partial dislocation may be left alone. When due to accident or disease it would better be removed.

CATARACT.

Opacity of the lens, or its capsule, or both, constitutes cataract. Numerous terms, which explain themselves, are used in classifying cataracts, such as lenticular, capsular and capsulo-lenticular; partial and complete; traumatic and spontaneous; fluid, soft and hard; congenital, juvenile and senile; immature, mature and hypermature; simple and complicated; stationary and progressive; gray, white, amber and black.

Cataracts are further classified by terms which indicate the location of the opacity as follows: —

1. **Anterior polar cataract**, in which the opacity is a small spot in the center of the anterior capsule, extending into the subjacent lens substance. It is usually pyramidal in shape, and may be congenital or acquired in early infant life. When congenital it is supposed to be the result of a fetal inflammation in which a deposit of lymph was left on the anterior capsule; or to be due to the adherence of the fetal pupillary membrane to the capsule. When acquired it is due to a perforation of the cornea which has allowed the lens to come forward in contact with the cornea.

2. **Posterior polar cataract**, similar to the preceding, except located in the center of the posterior capsule. In fetal life the hyaloid artery comes in contact with the lens at the posterior pole. An incomplete clearing up of the point of contact would explain a congenital posterior polar cataract. Another form of opacity generally called posterior polar but which in reality lies in the posterior cortex assumes the shape of a star or rosette; the center of the star corresponding to the posterior pole of the lens. It is usually associated with retinal or choroidal disease.

3. **Lamellar or zonular cataract**, in which the opacity is confined to one of the layers of the lens. It is assumed

that there is a disturbance of nutrition at a period of fetal life subsequent to the development of the clear nucleous. The layer of lens substance developed at the time of the nutritive disturbance is opaque. The interruption to the normal development of lens matter being temporary the subsequent layers are transparent.

4. Nuclear cataract in which the opacity begins in the hard center of the lens.

5. Cortical cataract, in which the opacity begins at the periphery of the lens.

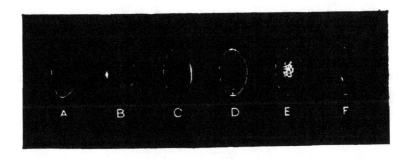

FIG. 82. — A, normal lens; B, anterior polar cataract; C, posterior polar cataract; D, cortical cataract; E, nuclear cataract; F, Lamellar cataract. (Juler.)

Symptoms. — In children, if the cataract is complete, it is easily diagnosed, as the pupillary area will be white or gray and the eye will be blind. If the cataract is zonular, which is the most frequent form in children, and is always congenital or arises in early infant life, the vision is much reduced, the child behaving as if near-sighted. Best vision is secured when the pupil is dilated, as the patient can then see around the opacity. Hence these children will shade their eyes or turn their backs to the light to get better vision, and will find their sight improved by the twilight or cloudy weather. Close inspection, with the pupil dilated, will reveal a pale, round, central opacity of the lens; the rim of the opacity being denser than the

center that will distinguish it from a nuclear cataract
which is denser in the center. It is often found that
children with zonular cataracts have been subject to infantile convulsions or are affected with rachitis. Anterior
polar cataract is easily detected by the small, snow-white
speck seen in the pupillary area. It does not affect vision
as much as the zonular variety. The great majority of
cataracts arise after the 45th year and are called senile.
They are usually nuclear or cortical. As a rule the first
symptom noticed is failing vision, not improved by glasses.
In some cases, in the first stages of the disease, the opacity
increases the index of refraction of the lens, and thus increases its refractive power sufficiently to enable the patient
to read without glasses. The patient rejoices in what is
commonly called *second sight.* Unfortunately this state is
temporary and gradual loss of vision follows. If the cataract is nuclear vision is improved by any circumstance
which dilates the pupil. There is generally some hyperemia of the conjunctiva, lacrymation and itching.
Sometimes inspection of the pupil reveals no anomaly, but
cataract, in the advanced stage, shows a distinct white or
grayish appearance of the pupillary area. Oblique focal
illumination will demonstrate some opacities, but to determine their presence in doubtful cases the ophthalmoscope
must be used. With the pupil dilated the whole lens can
be brought under inspection and the slightest opacity will
be detected by the opthalmoscope. The time between in-
cipiency and maturity varies greatly in different cases, and
in a few a partial opacity will remain stationary for the rest
of life. A traumatic cataract, due to rupture of the capsule, may swell so rapidly from imbibition of aqueous
humor as to bring on glaucomatous symptoms.

Cause. — Cataract is supposed to be due to some disturbance of the nutrition of the lens. It is a degenerative

change coming as do gray hairs, very little being known of the conditions that conduce to it. Diabetes, ergotism, heredity, glaucoma, hyperopia, and spasms in children are supposed to be etiological factors. Glass blowers, stokers, etc., whose eyes are exposed to excessive heat are supposed to be unusually subject to the disease. Traumatic cataracts are due to some accident which punctures the capsule or loosens the lens from its ligamentous attachment.

Treatment. — Spontaneous absorption of the cataract has been reported in a few authenticated cases, but no therapeutic agent has yet been discovered that will bring about this happy result. The treatment is surgical. For the operations suited to the different varieties consult a text book. Before operating or recommending a case for operation be sure to test the bad eye for other pathological conditions. Cataract prevents the distinction of objects, but does not obstruct light. Take the patient into a darkened room and with the good eye well covered see if he can point out the direction of a lighted candle when held in all parts of the field of vision. If he can readily follow the light his retina and optic nerve are healthy and a successful operation will make him see again. If he can not see the light at all an operation is useless. If he sees only in certain parts of the field, or detects slowly the difference between light and shadow, an operation will be proportionately meager of results.

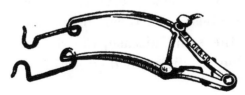

FIG. 83. — Speculum used to hold the lids open in operations upon the eyeball.

GLAUCOMA.

The vitreous and crystalline lens being non-vascular bodies, are nourished by lymph. This lymph is secreted by the choroid, the vascular part of the ciliary body and the posterior surface of the iris. The process of secretion being continuous, there must be a coincident excretion, and we find this takes place in the angle of the anterior chamber, through the spaces of Fontana, which connect with the canal of Schlemm. The direction of the current is from the vitreous, around the lens, into the posterior aqueous chamber, thence through the pupil into the anterior aqueous chamber, thence through the spaces of Fontana and canal of Schlemm into the anterior ciliary veins. Normal intra-ocular tension is dependent upon the maintenance of a physiological balance between the secretion and excretion of the aqueous humor.

The normal resistance of the globe, when palpated by the index finger of each hand, is designated by the letters Tn. If the globe is abnormally hard its increased tension is designated relatively by the signs T+?, T+1, T+2, and T+3. If abnormally soft, by T—?, T—1, T—2, and T—3.

Glaucoma is a diseased condition, due to excessive intra-ocular pressure. It may be idiopathic or secondary to some other pathological condition of the eye. Idiopathic or primary glaucoma may be simple or inflammatory. The inflammatory form is usually divided into acute, sub-acute, and chronic varieties. All forms of primary glaucoma are pathologically the same disease, the different aspects presented being due to different degrees of intensity. I will therefore give the symptoms of a mild form (simple glaucoma), and a severe manifestation (acute inflammatory glaucoma); it being understood that the disease may assume innumerable types, varying in intensity, between the two. It must be remembered that glaucoma is generally a disease of relapses and remissions which will always eventuate in total blindness.

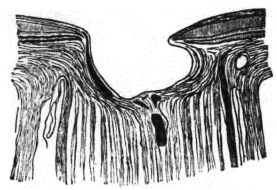

FIG. 84.— Section of very deep glaucoma cup. (Nettleship.)

Symptoms of simple glaucoma. — The patient will probably first notice a failure in vision for near work — an unnatural presbyopia, which will necessitate the use of convex lenses at an unusually early age, or require lenses stronger than the age of the patient would naturally demand. Artificial lights may be surrounded by halos or colored rings. At times a mist seems to obscure vision, and occasionally the patient will find himself in total darkness for several seconds. A slight dull pain of a neuralgic character may or may not be felt in and around the ball. The eye generally appears normal except for a slight dilatation of the pupil, the possible existence of an unusual whiteness of the sclera and the presence of a few large and tortuous conjunctival vessels. In the early stages visual acuity may or may not be reduced, but the field of vision will most likely show peripheral contraction, greatest on the nasal side, and scotoma may exist. Tension of the ball will be increased, with periodic variations in degree, at times approximating so closely to the normal that its glaucomatous nature may not be appreciable.

If the disease has existed for some time, the characteristic cupping or excavation of the optic disc will be seen. If tension is appreciably high, there may be spontaneous pulsation of the retinal arteries. Patients suffering with simple glaucoma often consult a physician *only* because vision is impaired and are unconscious of the presence of any pathological condition. Simple glaucoma may slowly deprive its victim of sight without manifesting any symptoms more active than those detailed, but it frequently changes into the inflammatory type. Simple glaucoma always attacks both eyes, but rarely at the same time. It sometimes occurs in young people and may be found in myopic eyes, which seem to be more or less immune to inflammatory glaucoma.

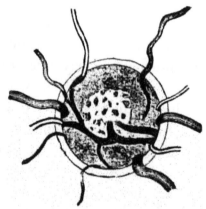

Fig. 85.—Ophthalmoscopic appearance of deep cupping of the disc in glaucoma. (Nettleship.)

Symptoms of acute inflammatory glaucoma.—The attack comes on suddenly and, as a rule, at night. It may or may not have been preceded by premonitory symptoms, such as failure of vision for near work, the presence of colored rings around lights, and temporary obscurations of sight. The true nature of the attack may be overlooked, owing to the severe pains in the head and face and the probable presence of an increase in pulse and temperature with vomiting. Tension of the globe is markedly increased, the lids edematous, the conjunctiva injected and chemotic. The cornea will be more or less opaque or steamy and anesthetic, the anterior chamber shallow and its contents possibly cloudy from the presence of lymphoid cells. The pupil will be widely dilated. The interior of the eye will probably not be visible, owing to the opacity of the cornea, but if the fundus can be viewed the veins will appear distended and sinuous and the arteries will be small and show pulsation. If glaucoma has not previously existed the disc will probably not be excavated but it will appear soon if the high tension continues.

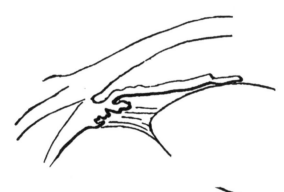

FIG. 86.—Angle of the anterior chamber in the normal eye. (Birnbacher.)

Vision will of course be greatly reduced. The symptoms may be so intense as to destroy the eye in a few hours in which case the disease is called *glaucoma fulminans.* As a rule, the symptoms abate and the eye may return almost to the normal in appearance, without however a return of the pre-existing visual acuity. After the lapse of a variable period another attack supervenes, resulting in an additional loss of vision, and so the disease progresses until the absolute state is established and blindness results.

In *absolute glaucoma* the ball is hard, pain constant and intense, the lens cataractous and pushed forward. The pupil is widely dilated and fixed. The sclera is bluish in color, with a dusky, red, circumcorneal zone, caused by engorgement of the anterior ciliary veins. The cornea is lustreless and vision — even light perception — is gone.

Further changes through which the eye may pass are *degenerative*. There may be ulceration of the cornea with perforation, followed by panophthalmitis and phthisis bulbi. The sclera may give way and staphyloma result; or the eye may slowly atrophy as a result of choroiditis, changes in the vitreous and detachment of the retina.

Cause. — In general terms hypersecretion or sub-normal excretion of the intra-ocular fluid are responsible for the train of symptoms called glaucoma. Blocking up the angle of the anterior chamber (Fig. 87) by diminishing excretion, is undoubtedly a potent factor in the production of the disease. The use of a mydriatic, by dilating the pupil, pushes the iris into the filtration angle, and will sometimes bring on an attack. The iris is supposed to be forced forward in such a way as to partially block the spaces of Fontana, when a large lens is associated with a small hyperopic eye. That this has something to do with the production of glaucoma seems plausible when we consider that the lens continues to grow until the 65th year and that about seventy per cent of all cases occur after the age of fifty and the same per cent are found in hyperopic eyes. An exacerbation may be excited by fatigue, grief, worry or anything which lowers vitality. Among the supposed etiological factors heredity, rheumatism and disturbances of circulation may be mentioned. Secondary glaucoma may be directly attributable to intra-ocular hemorrhage, complete anterior or posterior synechia, traumatic cataract with rapid swelling of the lens, intra-ocular tumors, etc.

Treatment. — As soon as positive of the diagnosis, do a broad iridectomy. This procedure is the most curative measure at our disposal. Though introduced in 1856 by Von Graefe, and practiced ever since that time, we do not yet know exactly how it produces the amelioration which

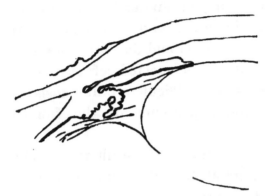

FIG. 87. — Angle of the anterior chamber in glaucoma closed by adhesion of iris-base to the periphery of the cornea. (Birnbacher.)

follows in the majority of cases. Removal of the superior cervical ganglion was introduced by Jonnesco. This procedure has not yet been subjected to a conclusive test. The medicinal treatment is practically limited to the use of the miotics, eserin and pilocarpin. The sulfate or salicylate of eserin is used in strength varying from $\frac{1}{4}$ to 2 grains to ʒi. Pilocarpin may be used twice as strong. The frequency of instillation is determined by their effect on the pupil. For the pain use hot fomentations and anodynes.

DISEASES OF THE RETINA.

HYPEREMIA AND ANEMIA.

The retinal vessels do not participate much in the changes of the intra-cranial circulation. There is some retinal congestion in meningitis and always venous engorgement in papillitis and thrombosis of a retinal vein. The same condition of the veins, in milder form, is often met with in emphysema and in weakness of the heart's action. Slight hyperemia of the retina and disc are sometimes associated with the strain of an uncorrected refractive error, but these mild hyperemias are difficult of diognosis owing to the variations in the appearance of the fundus, found in health.

Anemia of the retina may result from embolism of the central artery, great loss of blood, cholera, spasm of the arterial coats due to toxic doses of quinin and from spasm due to vaso-motor disturbance. The dimness of vision found in some cases of migraine or " blind headaches " are examples of the latter condition.

RETINAL CHANGE FROM DIRECT SUN RAYS; SNOW BLINDNESS; ELECTRIC OPHTHALMIA.

Persons who have looked directly at the sun have sometimes complained afterward of a central scotoma. These blind spots vary in their severity and persistency, sometimes being permanent. There may be central defect for colors, and also metamorphopsia. The ophthalmoscope will often show a minute lesion near the macula. The treatment consists of rest of eyes, dark glasses and hypodermatic injections of strychnin.

As a rule the only result, if any, of exposing the eyes to the glare of the snow is a mild form of conjunctivitis, but sometimes there is temporary, and, in rare instances, permanent amblyopia.

Exposure of the eyes to strong electric light, as in electric welding, may result in severe changes, such as are found in injury by direct sunlight, and may take a mild form of ophthalmia, such as is occasioned by exposure to snow. Electric workers now prevent these conditions by using glasses deeply colored with yellow, ruby or a combination of deep blue and red.

EMBOLISM AND THROMBOSIS OF RETINAL VESSELS.

Symptoms of Embolism.—Sudden loss of vision, partial if the obstruction lodges in a branch artery, total if it stops in the main trunk. The blood vessels will be much reduced in size. The retina will be white and opaque, the greatest opacity lying in the region around the macula and disc. The macula will appear as a cherry red spot, owing to the fact that it is much thinner than the rest of the retina, and the choroid shows through it. Degeneration of the retina occurs in a few days, soon followed by atrophy. The optic nerve generally atrophies. Vision is rarely restored.

Cause.—The plug may come from vegetations in the heart, due to valvular disease or endocarditis. It may also result from aneurism of the aorta or from atheroma of the arteries. It also occurs with Bright's disease and pregnancy.

Symptoms of Thrombosis.—The extent of visual loss depends upon the location of the thrombus in the central vein or one of its branches. Vision is, as a rule, not lost as suddenly as in embolism. There will be edema of the disc, tortuosity and engorgement of the veins, and numerous hemorrhages in the area drained by the thrombotic vein.

Cause.—Retarded venous circulation of the old, the emphysematous or those suffering with cardiac lesions. It may also be due to phlebitis.

Treatment of embolism and thrombosis is of little avail.

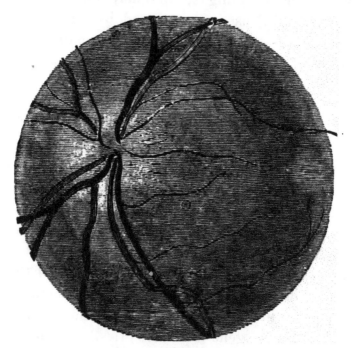

FIG. 88. — Serous or simple retinitis.   (Meyer.)

RETINITIS.

Inflammation of the retina may be limited to this membrane or may be associated with inflammation of the optic nerve (neuro-retinitis) or choroid (choroido-retinitis). The disc is usually involved unless the retinitis is very mild, and some opacity of the vitreous often co-exists. Owing to the fact that the disease is generally constitutional in origin, we find it almost always bilateral. Normally the retina is a transparent membrane, but when inflamed it appears smoky or hazy and, at times, to such an extent as to obscure its vessels in some part of their course. The veins may appear unusually large and tortuous and frequently there are hemorrhages. Often there will appear distinct white spots arranged along the course of the vessels or around the macula or disc. These spots can be differentiated from choroidal atrophy by the absence of the pigmented border and the softness of their outline. In retinitis there will be dimness of vision in all degrees.

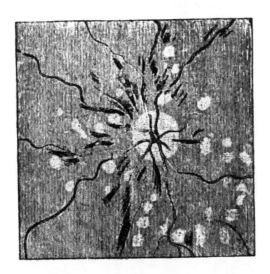

FIG. 89. — Recent severe retinitis in renal disease. (Gowers.)

There may be limitation of the field of vision and perhaps scotomata. Micropsia (objects appearing unnaturally small), megalopsia (objects unnaturally large), metamorphopsia (unnatural position of objects in the field, straight lines appearing wavy, etc.) and night blindness are forms of visual disturbance which may be manifested. There may be photophobia but there will be no pain and no external evidence of inflammation. Recovery may take

9

place with little or no loss of vision but generally the prognosis is grave. The result depends largely upon the cause of the attack, and the region of the retina involved. Different forms of the disease are named according to etiology, leukemic, albuminuric, diabetic, gouty and syphilitic. There are other forms named from characteristic features such as simple, hemorrhagic and purulent retinitis.

Albuminuric retinitis occurs in about seven per cent of all forms of albuminuria. It appears late in the stage of the renal trouble, the majority of patients dying within two years after its advent. Both eyes are generally affected. The characteristic feature is the presence of the white spots of fatty degeneration above described. Complete recovery from albuminuric retinitis has been observed.

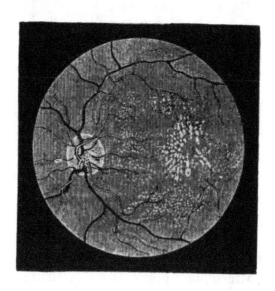

FIG. 90. — Renal retinitis at a late stage. (Wecker and Jaeger.)

Syphilitic retinitis occurs from congenital as well as acquired syphilis. It is, as a rule, associated with choroiditis and opacity of the vitreous. Night blindness is a prominent symptom. The general characteristics are those enumerated above witiout the wiite spots, wiici are almost patiognomonic of renal disease.

Cause. — Generally one of the constitutional conditions enumerated above is responsible for the disease. The etiology of simple, idiopatiic retinitis is obscure.

Treatment. —Demand absolute rest of the eyes. Subdue the ligit by the use of smoked glasses. Treat the constitution as indicated by eaci case.

RETINITIS PIGMENTOSA.

Tiis is a degenerative ratier tian an inflammatory condition. It is extremely cironic in its course, sometimes requiring years to reaci its usual termination in blindness.

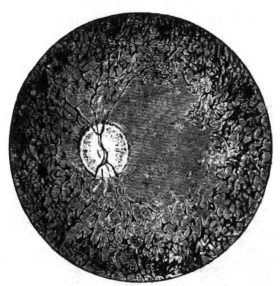

FIG. 91.—Pigmentary degeneration of the retina.   (Jaeger.)

Vision is much affected, but the symptom most complained of is nyctalopia (night blindness). The field of vision gradually contracts until only central vision is left. Tiis muci may remain for years. The fundus siows a peculiar stellate pigmentation beginning at its peripiery and extending gradually to the macula. The amount of pigment is no measure of the gravity of the case. The calibre of the retinal vessels diminishes and there is slow atrophy of the retina and disc, with occasional opacity of the posterior lens capsule.

The cause is obscure, but consanguinity of parents seems to be an etiological factor. No treatment is successful. Galvanism and strychnin have been recommended.

DETACHMENT OF THE RETINA.

This condition consists in a separation of the retina from the choroid, the intervening space being occupied by a serous fluid, blood or a tumor. Vision is affected in proportion to the extent and location of the detachment, the field showing a defect corresponding to the position of the lesion. The ophthalmoscope reveals a steel gray reflex from the detached part, over which the retinal vessels flow.

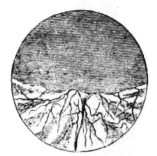

FIG. 92. — Ophthalmoscopic appearance of detached retina. (After Wecker and Jaeger.)

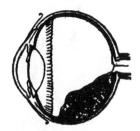

FIG. 93. — Section of eye with partial detachment of retina. (Nettleship.)

The presence of the vessels distinguishes this from any other condition presenting a similar reflex. If the detachment be recent there will be partial loss of vision, which increases with the degeneration of the retina. The retina rarely returns to its normal condition. The size of the detachment may remain stationary and may extend over the entire fundus.

Cause. — Blows u)on the ball or jars by transmitted force. Tumors of the cioroid. Disease resulting in fluidity or sirinkage of the vitreous. High degrees of myopia.

Treatment. — Iong continued rest in bed with eye bandaged. Evacuation of the subretinal fluid by a knife, needle or pointed cautery; or absor)tion of it by)ilocar)ine sweats and abstinence from fluids. The results of treatment are discouraging.

LESSON XXIII.

DISEASES OF THE OPTIC NERVE.

Optic Neuritis, or inflammation of the optic nerve, may be divided into two kinds: —

1. Papillitis, which involves the intra-ocular end of the nerve.

2. Retro-bulbar Neuritis, which affects the nerve between the ball and the chiasm.

PAPILLITIS.

The optic disc or papilla is the intra-ocular termination of the nerve or that part between the lamina cribrosa and the retina. With the ophthalmoscope the disc appears as a white circular area in the orange colored groundwork of the choroid. The white reflex of the disc is caused by the lamina cribrosa showing through the transparent nerve fibres. In inflammation of the disc there are no definite subjective signs. There is usually contraction of the field of vision and derangement of color perception, but vision may not be reduced until late in the progress of the disease. Main reliance in diagnosis is placed on the ophthalmoscope, which shows a serous infiltration of the disc manifested by redness, swelling and loss of its outline. The retinal arteries appear small and the veins filled and tortuous. The strangulation of the veins sometimes results in hemorrhages in the retina. In the great majority of cases both nerves are inflamed. If the inflammation extend by continuity of tissue to the retina, the condition is called *neuro-retinitis*. Papillitis may sometimes result in complete

.recovery, but in the majority of cases a partial or total atrophy of the nerve results.

Cause. — If monolateral it is generally the result of some orbital lesion. Wien bilateral it is usually due to intra-cranial disease, most frequently to tumors, but it may be due to meningitis, abscess, depressed fracture or softening.

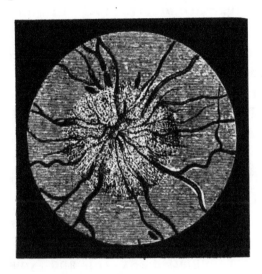

FIG. 94. — Appearance of a severe recent papillitis. Several elongated patches blood near the border of the disc. (Jackson.)

It may also be the result of albuminuria, diabetes, syphilis, lead poison and anemia. The prognosis will depend largely upon the etiology.

Treatment. — Forbid use of eyes. Direct your efforts to the cause, and wien in doubt give iodid of potassium, and build up the constitution by the usual metiods.

RETRO-BULBAR NEURITIS.

Tiis condition is also called central amblyopia and toxic amblyopia.

Symptoms. — Ioss of acute vision, the patient complaining of a mist before the eyes. Tiere will be central scotoma for red and green, and in advanced cases, central scotoma for objects. The affection is nearly always binocular and the vision of the two eyes nearly the same. There is no contraction of the field which aids in the differentiation from progressive atrophy. In pronounced cases, the disc shows an unnatural whiteness of its temporal side, and in an advanced state the whole disc may present the appearance of atrophy. There is proliferation of connective tissue in the nerve and atrophy of those fibres which go to the macula. The progress of the disease is slow, and the chance of recovery good unless of too long standing. It is almost exclusively a disease of men.

Cause. — It is due, in the great majority of cases, to the excessive use of tobacco or alcohol. Many observers consider tobacco the most potent etiological factor, and some entirely acquit alcohol of any responsibility for the disease. Alcoholic extract of Jamaica ginger is very popular in some prohibition regions and a number of serious cases of amblyopia have been reported from its use. Exposure to cold, diabetes, rheumatism, syphilis and poison by some chemicals, among which are iodoform and bisulfid of carbon, are supposed to be causative; and there are also some cases in which no cause can be discovered.

Treatment. — Absolute abstinence from the offending poison. Watch the patient's digestion and give iodid of potassium or strychnin.

QUININ AMBLYOPIA.

Overdoses of quinin cause another form of toxic amblyopia in which the symptoms are so different from those just enumerated, as to merit a separate description.

Symptoms. — The general symptoms of cinchonism will precede the loss of vision. The amount of visual disturbance varies from a blurring of objects to absence of light perception. The pupils may be widely dilated and the ophthalmoscope reveal a picture similar to that presented by embolism of the central artery. When there is sufficient vision to make a test possible, the field will be found contracted and color perception lost. After a variable period vision is decidedly improved though it rarely returns entirely to the normal. Salicylate of sodium and acetanilid can also produce a similar amblyopia.

Cause. — The action of the drug on the vaso-motor centers is supposed to be such as to cause a violent constriction of the blood vessels. An anemia of the retina is the result.

Treatment. — Use of the offending drug should be discontinued at once. Inhalations of nitrite of amyl may be tried. Strychnin should be given until constitutional effect is felt. Absolute rest of the eyes must be enforced and general health promoted in every way.

ATROPHY OF THE OPTIC NERVE.

In atrophy the medullary part of the fibres is displaced by granular fat and connective tissue, with thickening of the walls of the vessels and narrowing of their calibre.

Symptoms. — There is no pain and no change in the appearance of the ball, unless total blindness exists, when the pupils will be dilated. Great variety is manifested in the visual defects. The loss of vision may be rapid but is generally very gradual and slow. Central vision is lowered and the field contracts, sometimes concentrically, sometimes irregularly. Color sense becomes defective or lost, perception of green, red and blue usually disappearing in the order named. If the atrophy be associated with spinal cord lesions we shall, as a rule, find the Argyll-Robertson pupil. The disc will appear abnormally white or gray, slight excavation due to shrinkage of its substance may be noticed and the retinal vessels will be reduced in size.

Cause. — Spinal diseases of which tabes dorsalis is the most important, papillitis, pressure of tumors, disease of the orbit, thrombosis and embolism of the retinal vessels, glaucoma, meningitis, syphilis, alcoholism and anemia from great loss of blood may cause atrophy of the optic nerve. It may appear as a purely local disease independent of any other lesion.

Treatment. — Correct any derangement of general function. The galvanic current, one pole over the eye and the other at the back of the neck, is of doubtful utility. Give iodid of potassium, mercury or strychnin to the point of tolerance. Strychnin is more efficacious when given hypodermatically. Antipyrin, seven and a half grains every other day, hypodermatically is also recommended. Treatment is usually ineffectual.

FUNCTIONAL DISORDERS OF VISION, ETC.

AMBLYOPIA AND AMAUROSIS.

These are terms used to express a diminution or loss of vision without any apparent lesion. The two words are used, more or less indiscriminately, but amaurosis is generally applied to the graver conditions. There are many forms of lowered vision, the pathology of which is known, but they do not come under this head. The cause of functional amblyopia may be known but the exact way in which the loss of vision is produced is unexplained.

1. **Traumatism** to the head, direct or indirect, or a blow upon the eye, may be followed by amblyopia, more or less persistent. In these cases it is presumed that there is some invisible lesion of the parts concerned in vision.

2. **Loss of blood** may produce amblyopia, which probably is due to the fact that the retina is affected by the general lack of nutrition. But we do not know why the degree of amblyopia is not always commensurate with the amount of blood lost or why there is greater tendency to amblyopia from hemorrhages of the stomach, uterus and bowels than from traumatic hemorrhages.

3. **Congenital amblyopia** generally affects but one eye. It has been mentioned as a factor in the production of concomitant strabismus. It is supposed to be due to an arrest of development in fetal or early infant life. Lowered visual acuity is often associated with pronounced errors of refraction, especially astigmatism. If accurately

corrected at an early age the eye may gradually develop normal acuteness of vision.

4. **Hysterical amblyopia** may occur in both sexes but is most frequent in females. As might be supposed the symptoms assume a great variety of forms, such as total blindness, hemianopsia, scotoma, color blindness and contraction of the visual field. Neurasthenic school children, especially girls, are frequently thus afflicted and great tact and judgment are required in their treatment.

5. **Simulated amblyopia** or malingering, may be due to a desire to exaggerate an injury over which a lawsuit is pending, to secure a pension, to escape some disagreeable duty or to excite sympathy. For obvious reasons, but one eye is claimed to be affected. Numerous tests will reveal the patient's hypocrisy, if he claims blindness in but one eye, among which are the following: —

1. Put on him a pair of spectacles, one lens of which is plain glass and the other a prism with its base up or down. If malingering he will see double and an effort to walk, especially to go down stairs, will be made so cautiously that his true condition is detected.

2. Place before the eye he claims is bad a plain glass and before the other a plus glass just strong enough to obscure its vision. If with these, vision is normal, the patient is malingering.

3. Hang some green letters in front of a *black* background, at a convenient distance. Hold before the good eye a glass colored red. If he reads the letters, he does it with his bad eye as the green letters cannot be seen through the red glass. Red letters on a *white* background can not be seen through a red glass.

4. Put a drop or two of atropin in the good eye and to allay suspicion an equal number of drops of cocain may be put in the bad eye. When time enough has elapsed for

the atropin to paralyze accommodation and, the patient
a book. If he reads it he does so with the eye he claims
to be amblyopic.

If the patient claims to be blind in both eyes his detection is more difficult and a close watch may be necessary to
determine the true condition. A simple test, which may
be of service, is to ask the patient to look at his own hand.
A blind man will turn the eyeballs toward the hand, a
malingerer may intentionally look in some other direction.

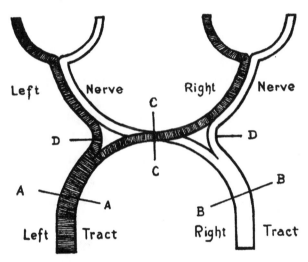

FIG. 95.—Lesion at A, A, would cause right homonymous hemianopsia. B, B,
would cause left homonymous hemianopsia. C, C, would cause bitemporal hemianopsia. D, D, would cause binasal hemianopsia.

HEMIANOPSIA.

Hemianopsia is a term used to express diminution or total
loss of vision in one-half of the field. Both eyes are usually
affected, which indicates a lesion in or back of the chiasm.
If only one eye is affected the lesion is probably in front of
the chiasm. In the great majority of cases of hemianopsia
affecting both eyes the diminution or loss of vision will be
in the right half of each field or the left half of each field.

This is called *homonymous* hemianopsia. We may have loss of the external half of each field called *bitemporal* hemianopsia, or of the internal half of each field called *binasal* hemianopsia, but these conditions are rare. A condition still more uncommon is loss of the upper or lower field. The lesion which causes hemianopsia may lie at any part of the visual tract from the eyeball to the cortex of the brain and a knowledge of the origin and distribution of the optic nerve fibres is necessary to determine its location. The lesion may be a tumor, periostitis, blood clot, softening of the brain, atheroma of adjacent vessels, injuries, etc. Treatment must be directed to the cause.

NYCTALOPIA OR NIGHT BLINDNESS.

Most authors use the word hemeralopia to express night blindness and nyctalopia to express day blindness. Green-hill has proven that they are in error and that the reverse is correct according to derivation and ancient usage. The night blindness of retinitis pigmentosa must not be confounded with the *functional* variety being described in which there are no visible lesions of the fundus. In functional night blindness vision may be normal in a bright light but is greatly lowered on dull days, in the twilight or in dimly lighted rooms. It is found in persons who have been exposed to glaring light, such as travelers in the tropics, glass blowers, electric welders and those who work before furnaces. It is also supposed to be associated with certain states of lowered vitality such as scorbutus, starvation, etc.

The treatment consists in protection of the eyes by dark glasses, the use of tonics of quinin, iron, strycnin and cod liver oil, and changing the occupation if that seems at fault.

HEMERALOPIA OR DAY BLINDNESS.

This condition is the opposite to nyctalopia in that the patient sees better and greatly prefers diminished illumination. It is found as a symptom in retro-bulbar neuritis, albinism, dilatation of the pupil from third nerve paralysis or from the use of a mydriatic, central cataract, etc. It also exists as a *functional* condition independent of any demonstrable lesion. Functional hemeralopia is found in persons who have been excluded from the light for a long period and is also a frequent symptom of hysteria.

When hemeralopia is a symptom, the primary affection should be treated. If it is functional examine closely for muscular insufficiency and errors of refraction; build up the constitution and accustom the eyes to light by resorting to the strategy demanded by each case.

DIAGNOSTIC TABLE.

	CONJUNCTIVITIS.	INTERSTITIAL KERATITIS.	IRITIS.	ACUTE GLAUCOMA.
Redness.	Palpebral and ocular conjunctiva injected. Pericorneal zone the last part to get red.	Pericorneal zone injected. In bad cases the entire ocular conjunctiva becomes red.	Pericorneal zone injected first, entire ocular conjunctiva liable to become congested.	Diffuse redness with conjunctival chemosis and edema of the lid.
Pain.	Burning and scratchy as if there was a foreign body in eye.	Generally slight, but in some cases severe.	Sometimes absent but usually severe, following the fifth nerve into the cheek and forehead.	Always severe, following the fifth nerve into the cheek and forehead.
Vision.	Unimpaired or slightly diminished by mucus on the cornea.	Greatly diminished and same in all parts of the field of vision.	Diminished by turbidity of the aqueous humor but not as bad as in interstitial keratitis or acute glaucoma.	Greatly diminished; nasal side of field first and most.
Discharge.	Muco-purulent or purulent.	Watery.	Watery and profuse.	Watery.

Tenderness on pressure.	None.	None.	Slight. Considerable over the ciliary body if it be involved.	Great.
Tension.	Normal.	Normal.	Possibly slightly increased.	Greatly increased.
Temperature, pulse, etc.	Normal.	Normal.	Normal.	Increase in temperature and pulse, sometimes vomiting.
Cornea.	Normal.	Hazy, pink or buff colored sometimes hyper-sensitive.	Normal.	Hazy, with sub-normal sensitiveness.
Age of patient.	Any.	Disease of childhood, rarely seen after 25 years.	Any age, but rare before puberty.	Rarely seen in patients under 35.

10

INDEX.

tezone grs ½
ar drst Ʒi
: Every 4 hrs. Eye Wash. — Purulent Discharge